Word Formation and Transparency in Medical English

Word Formation and Transparency in Medical English

Edited by

Pius ten Hacken and Renáta Panocová

Cambridge Scholars Publishing

Word Formation and Transparency in Medical English

Edited by Pius ten Hacken and Renáta Panocová

This book first published 2015

Cambridge Scholars Publishing

Lady Stephenson Library, Newcastle upon Tyne, NE6 2PA, UK

British Library Cataloguing in Publication Data
A catalogue record for this book is available from the British Library

ISBN (10): 1-4438-8002-7
ISBN (13): 978-1-4438-8002-2

TABLE OF CONTENTS

List of Illustrations

LIST OF TABLES

INTRODUCTION

MEDICAL LANGUAGE, WORD FORMATION AND TRANSPARENCY

PIUS TEN HACKEN AND RENÁTA PANOCOVÁ

As a side effect of the rapid progress in medical research and of the emergence of new medical conditions, medicine is a domain where new concepts have to be named more frequently than in many other domains. Because of the prominent position of English in medical research, most of these new concepts are first named in English. This volume takes this situation as a background for the study of naming strategies used for such new concepts. Before introducing the individual chapters, in this introduction we will present some general thoughts about the nature of medical language, the role of word formation in naming, and the question of what constitutes transparency.

1 Medical language

A first question to be asked in a volume devoted to medical language is what kind of language is designated by the expression *medical language*. In English, we use the adjective *English* as a noun when it refers to the language. In Slavic languages, this is not common. Thus, in Polish one rather finds *język angielski* ('language English', i.e. the English language) than just *angielski* ('English') to refer to the language. However, for specialized languages, we cannot leave out the noun in English. We cannot use *medical* to mean *medical language*. This provides a first indication that *medical language* is not perceived as a language in the same way as *English*.

For a long time, linguists assumed that English, Dutch, Slovak, and other languages should be taken as the basic objects of study in linguistics. In 19th century historical-comparative linguistics, the historical development of such objects and their relationships were taken as central.

Thus, August Schleicher (1821-1868) proposed a genealogical tree of Indo-European languages (cf. Collinge 1995: 198). With his distinction between synchronic and diachronic linguistics, Saussure (1916) changes the emphasis, focusing more on the state of such languages at a particular point in time than on their development and relations, but he maintains the idea of a language as an object of study. A question that was not systematically pursued was how we can establish whether a language in fact has a particular property. What is the empirical basis for the claims that English has no grammatical gender, Dutch has a phonemic contrast between /f/ and /v/, and Slovak has seven nominal cases?

A central insight into the nature of language is Chomsky's (1965: 4) distinction between *competence* and *performance*. As explained in more detail in ten Hacken (2007: 42-46), both competence and performance are empirical objects, the former the knowledge of language of an individual speaker as realized in the speaker's brain, the latter the utterances and texts produced applying this knowledge. As argued by ten Hacken (2007: 274-281), it was only in the course of the 1970s that Chomsky realized that in this model there was no place for languages such as English. Some of the properties that we ascribe to English are clearly not compatible with competence and performance. Thus, English is the language of the UK, the USA, and a number of other countries. It is one of the drafting languages of the EU. It is the language of Chaucer, Shakespeare, Jane Austen and J.K. Rowling. It has been spoken since the 6th century CE. In the sense in which *English* has such properties, it is not an empirical object. We can only arrive at a notion of *English* by classifying linguistic knowledge (i.e. speakers) or linguistic output (i.e. texts and utterances).

This insight changes the way in which a claim such as the one that English has no grammatical gender can be tested. We can determine whether this claim holds for English as competence only to the extent that we narrow down the scope of the claim to an individual speaker. For English as performance, we can test the claim for a particular corpus of texts and utterances. For English as a language, it is not possible even in principle to collect direct empirical evidence. We can only approach the question either by first determining that a speaker or a set of speakers is characteristic of English and then study their competence or by first collecting a corpus to which we assign the label that it is representative of English and study its properties. In both cases, we take decisions that are not determined by the data before we can do any empirical investigation. English is not an empirical object.

Medical language differs from English in several ways. It is not a natural question, for instance, to ask whether someone speaks medical language, as opposed to the question whether someone speaks English. Medical language is also language-specific. English medical language differs from Dutch or Slovak medical language. This raises the question of the relationship between English medical language and English, but also of the relationship with Dutch and Slovak medical language.

A framework that has often been used as a basis for approaching such questions is that of sublanguages. Here, the idea is that English medical language is a sublanguage of English. The original idea of sublanguages stems from Harris (1968). Kittredge (1987: 59-60) defines a sublanguage L_S as a subsystem of a language L, such that L_S is part of L, but has a more restricted domain and community of speakers. L_S is a consistent and complete linguistic system, so that it has its own sets of vocabulary items and syntax rules. Kittredge proposes to derive them from the analysis of a corpus. It is fairly straightforward to do this for the vocabulary. For the grammar rules, Kittredge (1987: 62-63) makes the following observations:

> First, in a sublanguage, the rules for constructing meaningful sentences can be made much more precise than in the language as a whole. These rules can be related in terms of word classes which are discovered by studying the distributional properties of words in texts. Second, in a sublanguage the rules for constructing sentences may be quite different from (and even contrary to) the rules for sentences in the 'standard' language.

For medical English, this means that we have to collect a corpus of texts as a preliminary. In compiling such a corpus, we have to take decisions. The corpus is of course an empirical object, but the decision whether a text belongs to medical English is based on a judgement, not on any empirical fact. A crucial question seems to be whether the corpus as a whole is representative of English medical language. However, there is no way to go beyond intuitive judgements for answering this question.

In our view, it would be misguided to conclude from this argument that the concept of *medical English* should not be used. Otherwise we would not edit a volume that has *medical English* in its title. An important observation in this respect is that not all concepts we evoke in an academic text have to be precisely delimited terms. Although Chomsky often made the point that there is no object called *English*, Chomsky & Lasnik (1995: 33) state that "[i]n English, generally only objective Case-assigning verbs can occur in the passive". The use of *English* in this quotation is not incoherent with the observation that there is no such object. In this quotation, English is used pretheoretically.

In the same way we can make statements about medical English, without implying that there is an entity called *medical English* for which the statement is correct. However, we cannot determine, for example, the exact number of words in medical English. In this volume, *medical English* will be used as a pretheoretical notion. We do not make any claims that depend on the precise boundaries of the concept.

2 Word formation

Word formation is a system of rules that can produce new words on the basis of existing lexical items. Word formation can be distinguished from syntax. Both take lexical items as their input, but whereas syntax produces sentences to express thoughts, word formation produces words to name concepts. Word formation has an onomasiological function and changes the lexicon.

In medical language, word formation is particularly prominent because there is a steady growth in the number of concepts that need to be named. For the study of word formation this naming need is important, because it is a decisive factor in activating word formation. Only when there is a new concept that needs a name will word formation rules be activated. However, naming needs can also be fulfilled in other ways. The most prominent alternative naming procedures are sense extension and borrowing.

An example of sense extension in medical English is the use of *cell* for a small unit of the body. The original meaning was a small room in a monastery or prison. This example shows how sense extension is based on metaphoric or metonymic sense relationships. It also illustrates the notion of *onomasiological coercion*. Much of the meaning of the resulting term is determined by the concept we started with, independently of the naming mechanism and the input. That a cell has a nucleus and multiplies by fission cannot be derived from *cell* in the sense of a small room.

Given the large degree of international exchange in the field of medicine, it is not surprising that borrowing plays an important role as a naming mechanism. At the level of research, where new concepts are discovered and named, Latin used to be the language of international communication. Often, also Ancient Greek words were used in their Latinized form. By the time medicine went through the transition from a craft-like practice to an applied science, which as Bynum (1994) argues occurred in the 19th century, most medical research was no longer published in Latin. However, for the naming of new concepts Latin and Greek continued to be used in the form of neoclassical word formation. Especially at the time when several major European languages were used for international scientific communication, the use of neoclassical formations that could be recognized equally in each of these languages was a useful aid to understanding.

In the current situation, the overwhelming majority of medical research is published in English. As opposed to fields such as astronomy or mathematics, however, for communication in the field of medicine there is much more pressure to accommodate a wide range of other languages. This is because in medicine there is always a need to communicate in vernacular languages of the communities. Medical communication is not limited to researchers, but also includes patients and their relatives. At some point in the chain between researcher and patient, the terminology has to be translated. Here the question arises whether an English name should be borrowed or a language-specific alternative naming device used instead.

It is in this configuration that word formation operates. As opposed to alternative naming mechanisms, word formation is based on the application of rules. At the same time, in common with other naming mechanisms and in contrast to syntax, word formation is not rule-driven. The starting point is not a form and meaning determined by a word formation rule, but the need to name a specific concept. Word formation rules constrain the meaning of their output, but it is in general not fruitful to start from the word formation rule in trying to explain the full meaning of the resulting word. As argued by ten Hacken (2013), a much more promising approach is to start from the concept to be named. On the basis of this concept, a word formation rule and an input to this rule are chosen, but the full meaning only arises through onomasiological coercion. This process can be illustrated on the basis of (1).

(1) cuvette oximeter

In (1), we have a compound consisting of the head *oximeter* and the non-head *cuvette*. The head looks like a neoclassical word formation, but in fact, *oxi* stands for *oxygen*, not for the Ancient Greek ὀξύς [oxys] ('sharp'). An oximeter is an instrument for measuring the quantity of oxygen in blood. The non-head is a loanword from French. At the point where (1) is formed, *oximeter* and *cuvette* are words in the lexicon. The meaning of a compound is underspecified. We can deduce from the form that (1) designates a kind of oximeter that is related to (a) cuvette, but in order to understand the meaning in more detail we have to know the concept for which it was coined as a name. Stedman (1990) gives the meaning as in (2).

(2) an o[ximeter] that reads the percentage of oxygen saturation of the blood as it passes through a cuvette outside the body

The definition in (2) is given in a run-on entry to *oximeter*, which explains the abbreviation of this word. Significantly, the definition is almost entirely a description of the relation between the head and the non-head in (1).

Word formation rules are used to produce new words. This is not restricted to the speaker who uses this word for the first time in the language. First of all, it is hardly possible to determine which speaker used (1) for the first time. Secondly, the notion of *language* in "for the first time in the language" is the non-empirical, pretheoretical sense of language, of which we cannot determine the precise boundaries. However, every speaker coming across (1) and not having this word in their mental lexicon will use a word formation rule to interpret it. Depending on the speaker's needs, the word can then be stored in their lexicon or not. The meaning associated with (1) depends on the speaker's knowledge of and experience with the concept.

3 Transparency

There are different concepts that can be used to describe the relationship between the form and meaning of words. *Transparency* should be distinguished from *motivation* and *iconicity*. All of them contrast with Saussure's (1916: 100) statement in (3).

(3) Le lien unissant le signifiant au signifié est arbitraire[1]

Saussure gives the example of French *bœuf* ('ox') and its German translation *Ochs*. If (3) did not hold, we would have to find an explanation why not all languages have the same word for the same concept. Saussure (1916: 101) clarifies that *arbitraire* in (3) does not mean that any speaker can choose a *signifiant* at will, but that the form is "*immotivé*" ('unmotivated'), i.e. there is no natural link between the form and the meaning.

Whereas the existence of onomatopoeia is at best a marginal counterexample to (3), Saussure (1916: 180-184) modifies the scope of (3) somewhat in view of morphological relationships. He distinguishes

[1] 'The link uniting the signifier (i.e. the form) to the signified (i.e. the meaning) is arbitrary' [our translation, PtH & RP]

absolute and relative arbitrariness, so that, for instance, *happy* and *sad* are fully arbitrary, but *unhappy* is only partially arbitrary.

As indicated by the use of *immotivé*, the opposite of *arbitrary* for Saussure is rather *motivated* than *transparent*. In addition, we have the term *iconicity*, used in a similar way. However, there are different shades of meaning involved and it is worth distinguishing them. In explaining the contrast, we use the compound (1) as an example. The degree of motivation concerns the extent to which the speaker is guided to use this expression for the instrument it refers to. One of the decisions involved is the one to use a compound.

The degree of transparency concerns the extent to which the reader or hearer is helped by the form in the task of determining the meaning. Given that compounds in English are regularly right-headed, a reader will understand (1) as the name of a kind of oximeter. In this sense, compounding makes (1) more transparent than a non-compound might be, in particular a simple expression that is not the result of word formation. The underspecification of the relation between the head and non-head, however, reduces the transparency.

In the discussion of iconicity, neither the role of the speaker nor of the hearer is taken into account. As Dressler (2005: 268) states, the concept of *icon* is based on work by Charles S. Peirce (1839-1914). In the context of natural morphology, Mayerthaler (1981: 23) introduces *konstruktioneller Ikonismus* ('constructional iconicity'). The general idea is that more complex concepts have longer names. This applies to (1) in the sense that *cuvette oximeter* refers to a more specific type of instrument than *oximeter*.

In natural morphology, iconicity is connected to two related concepts, diagrammaticity and biuniqueness. Dressler (2005: 269) gives compounds as a typical example of diagrammaticity, because the semantic head is also the morphosyntactic head. A compound such as (1) is diagrammatic to the extent that its head *oximeter* determines at the same time the meaning, in the sense that (1) designates a type of oximeter, and the syntactic properties, to the extent that (1) is a countable noun like *oximeter*. Whereas iconicity is more of a quantitative notion, based on the amount of information, diagrammaticity concerns the relative contribution of morphological elements.

By biuniqueness, the one-to-one correspondence between form and meaning is meant. As noted by Dressler (2005: 274), this is particularly important in terminology. In classical approaches such as Wüster (1991), biuniqueness is almost axiomatic. However, as Dressler notes, it is only aimed for on a domain-internal basis. The fact that *induction* is used in medicine for the artificial stimulation of child birth but in mathematics for a particular type of proof is not problematic. Together, iconicity, diagrammaticity and biuniqueness can be used to describe the way in which meaning and form relate to each other without referring to a speaker or a hearer.

The three terms of *motivation*, *transparency*, and *iconicity* have not always been distinguished consistently in the literature. However, as far as we can judge, where two or three of them have been used in a contrastive sense, *motivation* is usually connected to the speaker perspective, *transparency* to the hearer perspective, and *iconicity* to a perspective that focuses on words as abstract objects. For *iconicity*, this means that it is independent of competence and performance, which in our view makes it a less interesting property for the study of the role and effects of word formation in medical English. The question of motivation is especially relevant in studies of productivity, an issue that is not central in this volume. It is therefore natural here, in our opinion, to make transparency the focus of the study of how word formation interacts with the relationship between form and meaning.

4 Overview of chapters

Our volume consists of eight chapters that can be divided into two parts of four chapters each. The first part concentrates on the study of transparency from a monolingual perspective; the second part contains studies of translation.

In chapter 1, Rachel Bryan focuses on International Nonproprietary Names (INNs) for pharmaceutical substances. In this context, transparency has a particular significance, because the names of the substances are used to identify the correct medical treatment for particular patients. Therefore, the World Health Organization (WHO) has elaborated a set of guidelines for arriving at an INN that is at the same time maximally transparent and sufficiently distinct. Bryan investigates how these guidelines are used in practice and to what extent they achieve their goals. One of the special features of INNs is that they are composed of formatives that have been assigned a meaning rather than on a system of word formation that has emerged naturally in a language.

In chapter 2, by Pilar León-Araúz, we turn to the psychiatric domain. She investigates the correlation between terminological variation and transparency. In the psychiatric domain, there are many synonyms that are distinguished in various ways. On one hand, there is a variety of registers ranging from formal to colloquial. These registers often correlate with the type of participants in the oral or written communication. On the other hand there are connotative factors that may make certain expressions more accessible or less acceptable. León-Araúz describes how a database to account for this variation is structured and gives some results that have been found by analysing the occurrence of variants in a specially constructed corpus.

In chapter 3, Pius ten Hacken takes an approach that can be characterized as corpus-based and semasiological in the sense that he studies the medical terminology used in a single text. This text is Gersdorff & Gérard's (2011) *Atlas of Middle Ear Surgery*, an introduction to a specialized area of medicine, written for otologists. Ten Hacken classifies the terms extracted from this text along morphological criteria and analyses how properties of the word formation rules involved affect the transparency of the terms. In his collection of terms, there is a large preponderance of compounds.

Chapter 4, by Renáta Panocová, delimits the domain of study more in a morphological way than on the basis of the medical specialization. As observed above, neoclassical word formation is an important source of terms in the medical domain. Even though nowadays few medical researchers have a sufficient command of Ancient Greek and Latin to write texts in these languages, neoclassical elements are still commonly used to name new medical concepts. Panocová compares the transparency of such formations with the transparency of some commonly used alternatives, in particular eponyms and abbreviations.

With chapter 5, we enter the second part of the volume, with studies involving translation. This chapter, written by Nina Patton, María Fernández Parra and Rocío Pérez Tattam, delimits the domain in morphological terms, looking at nominal compounds. There are two language pairs involved, English-Spanish and English-Slovak. A major challenge of these language pairs is that Spanish and Slovak do not have an immediately corresponding construction for English compounds. The authors investigate which constructions are used in the translation of English compounds in each language and to what extent the choice of construction is influenced by the relation between the head and the non-head of the English compound.

In chapter 6, Sevda Pekcoşkun takes a different perspective of translation. Her language pair is English-Turkish and her first question is which translation strategies are used in the translation of popular medical texts. Whereas for research articles in medicine, we can expect that many readers will put up with an English version in which they recognize many of the terms immediately as borrowings or internationalisms, for popular medical texts, it is important that Turkish speakers can read and understand them. This leads to Pekcoşkun's second question, where the influence of the choice of translation strategy on the intelligibility for the target readership is investigated. She uses questionnaires, asking readers to compare how easy different translations are for understanding.

The last two chapters study the language pair English-Polish. In chapter 7, by Mariusz Górnicz, the perspective is that of medical specialists and how they render English terminology in Polish. Górnicz argues that there is a strong resistance not only to borrowing English terms in Polish, but also to adopting the same structures in Polish as in English. A central concept in this context is what he calls *compression*, i.e. the techniques that lead to a more concise expression, so that terms are more efficient in communication than full descriptive phrases.

Finally, in chapter 8, Szymon Machowski returns once more to compounds. His research focuses on the domain of infectious diseases and he applies a classification based on two independent features. On one hand, he introduces four semantic categories and on the other, four formal properties of the expression. He then considers how English terms in these different categories are translated into Polish.

Most contributions to this volume are based on presentations at the Seminar 'Word formation and transparency in Medical English', organized by the editors at the 12th Conference of the European Society for the Study of English (ESSE) in Košice. We would like to thank all participants to this seminar who gave comments and asked questions, triggering a lively discussion that led to a better formulation of the ideas presented. We would also like to thank Sam Baker of Cambridge Scholars Publishing for suggesting the idea to edit a volume based on this workshop. In the production of this volume, we were helped by the very responsive authors who helped us to realize this idea. In producing the manuscript, we benefited from editorial support by Christina Muigg and proofreading by David Galvin.

We hope that the volume will be useful for medical text writers and translators in that it offers a range of perspectives on problems that they have to solve every day. At the same time, terminologists will find here a number of case studies. Morphologists, especially those working on word formation, may benefit from the study of naming practices in a number of areas that are related in the sense that they are all in the field of medicine, yet quite different in their actual approach to naming.

References

Bynum, W.F. (1994), *Science and the Practice of Medicine in the Nineteenth Century*, Cambridge: Cambridge University Press.

Chomsky, Noam (1965), *Aspects of the Theory of Syntax*, Cambridge (Mass.): MIT Press.

Chomsky, Noam & Lasnik, Howard (1995), 'The Theory of Principles and Parameters', in Chomsky, Noam, (ed.), *The Minimalist Program*, Cambridge, MA: MIT Press, pp. 13-127.

Collinge, N.E. (1995), 'History of Comparative Linguistics', in Koerner & Asher (eds.), *Concise history of the language sciences from the Sumerians to the cognitivists*, Oxford, pp. 195-202.

Dressler, Wolfgang U. (2005), 'Word-Formation in Natural Morphology', in Štekauer, Pavol & Lieber, Rochelle (eds.), *Handbook of Word-Formation*, Dordrecht: Springer, pp. 267-284.

Gersdorff, Michel & Gérard, Jean-Marc (2011), *Atlas of Middle Ear Surgery*, Stuttgart: Thieme.

ten Hacken, Pius (2007), *Chomskyan Linguistics and its Competitors*, London: Equinox.

—. (2013), 'Semiproductivity and the place of word formation in grammar', in ten Hacken, Pius & Thomas, Claire (eds.), *The Semantics of Word Formation and Lexicalization*, Edinburgh: Edinburgh University Press, pp. 28-44.

Harris, Zellig (1968), *Mathematical Structures of Language*, New York: Interscience.

Kittredge, Richard I. (1987), 'The significance of sublanguage for automatic translation', in Nirenburg, Sergei (ed.), *Machine Translation: Theoretical and Methodological Issues*, Cambridge: Cambridge University Press, pp. 59-67.

Mayerthaler, Willi (1981), *Morphologische Natürlichkeit*, Wiesbaden: Athenaion.

Saussure, Ferdinand de (1916), *Cours de linguistique générale*, Charles Bally & Albert Sechehaye (eds.), Édition critique préparée par Tullio de Mauro, Paris: Payot, 1981.

Stedman (1990), *Stedman's Medical Dictionary*, 25th edition, Hensyl, William R. (ed.), Baltimore: Williams & Wilkins.

Wüster, Eugen (1991), *Einführung in die allgemeine Terminologielehre und terminologische Lexikographie*, Bonn: Romanistischer Verlag.

CHAPTER ONE

TAXONOMY AND TRANSPARENCY IN INTERNATIONAL PHARMACEUTICAL NOMENCLATURE

RACHEL BRYAN

The language of medicine, although highly specialised, has a broad usership comprising multiple strata of the population with varying levels of knowledge for multiple purposes. This usership includes general practitioners, consultants, nurses, pharmacists, patients, parents and caregivers. No single person holds a comprehensive knowledge of every area and so there is great variation in understanding of the terminology and the degree to which its use is specialised. Medication names such as *morphine*, *Benadryl*, *paracetamol* and *adrenaline* surround us in our daily lives and are an important and under-researched area of terminology.

In antiquity, medications were named after the gods, e.g. morphine after Morpheus, the god of dreams and anandamide after Sanskrit *ananda*, 'bliss, delight' (OED). In the present day, pharmaceutical substances are named within a complex system of nomenclature which is managed by multiple government bodies. As illustrated in Figure 1-1, a pharmaceutical substance such as salbutamol (an asthma medication) will have three types of name.

- One chemical name, based upon the chemical formula of the substances, indicating the position of hydroxy groups, the length of the carbon chain and so on. This name is designated by the International Union of Pure and Applied Chemistry (IUPAC) and is published multilingually. There are some interesting translation problems in this area, but they are beyond the scope of this chapter.
- At least one brand, or proprietary name, chosen by the manufacturer that originally created the substance. This name is commercially driven, initially capitalized and legally bound to not imply any

therapeutic benefit. It is typically laconic and euphonious. Once out of patent (up to 20 years in the EU), the substance can be marketed by other companies and so will be assigned more brand names.

- At least one generic or non-proprietary name. On a global level, it will be assigned an International Nonproprietary Name (INN) by the World Health Organization (WHO), and in each country in which it is approved for use, it will be assigned a national generic name, such as a British Approved Name (BAN) in the UK, or a *Denominazione Comune Italiana* (DCIT) in Italy.

Chemical name	(*RS*)-4-[2-(*tert*-butylamino)-1-hydroxyethyl]-2-(hydroxymethyl)phenol formula: $C_{13}H_{21}NO_3$
Generic names	International Nonproprietary Name: salbutamol British Approved Name: salbutamol United States Adopted Name: albutamol
Proprietary names	Ventolin, Aerolin, Ventorlin, Asthalin, Proventil, ProAir

Fig. 1-1. The pharmacopoeial monograph for salbutamol[1]

1 International Nonproprietary Names

This chapter presents a qualitative analysis of the International Nonproprietary Name (INN) nomenclature, focusing in particular on the underlying conceptual taxonomy and semantic transparency. INNs will be the focus of this study as they are the most commonly used system of generic names, and their form is used by default in both the UK and the EU with only a few notable exceptions (Aronson 2000). There are over 8,000 INNs currently in use. INNs are designated by the WHO and are formally placed in the public domain to promote consistency of global communications between manufacturers, clinicians, prescribers and patients. The nomenclature is published in seven languages (WHO 1997). Given their international status, the name designation process in place must encompass a broad conceptual system and naming guidelines must be robust and stringently applied.

INNs are designated according to a set of guidelines (WHO 1997), which aim to achieve usability (pronounceable, legible, audibly perceptible, comprehensible and memorable), clarity (free from confusion)

[1] A pharmacopoeial monograph is a single document describing the name(s) and chemical formula of a pharmaceutical substance.

and taxonomy (showing relationship within the conceptual system). The WHO dictates that pharmacological relationship be shown by using a common 'stem', which may be a prefix, infix, suffix, or a 'freefix', and which can appear anywhere in the name. A 'stem' in this context is a word part to which a particular pharmacological meaning has been assigned and which is used to signify the relationship between substances. By using a common stem, substances are placed into pharmacological groups, related by anatomical target, therapeutic action, or chemical composition. The use of stems creates a taxonomic conceptual system for INNs and allows users to exploit this systematicity to increase retention, pronunciation and recognition of the names.

The INN programme began in 1952 and between 120 and 150 new names are designated each year. They are first created in Latin and this form is translated into the six official languages of the United Nations: English, French, Spanish, Russian, Chinese and Arabic. The Latin form of the name is used as the basis for translation into other European languages, such as Italian and Portuguese (Marecková *et al.* 2002).

Morphosemantic analysis of INNs is possible because their meaning is highly compositional, i.e. meaning is derived from the meanings of constituent parts (Deléger *et al.* 2009). In contrast to medical terminology in anatomy and general medicine, INNs are not full neoclassical compounds in that they cannot be parsed into elements directly derived from classical languages. INNs are composed of a random element, normally a prefix, and at least one stem. Stems are formed from three types of component. These types are listed in (1).

(1) a. abbreviations, such as the sub-stem *-tu-* in *situximab* denoting targeting tumorous tissue, or the stem *-kin* in *ilodecakin* denoting interleukin-type substances;
b. acronyms, such as the stem *-mab* in *urtoxazumab* denoting monoclonal antibodies; and
c. elements of chemical nomenclature. These can be seen as adapted neoclassical forms, such as the stem *-fos* (from Latin *phosphorous*) in *clofenvinfos*, denoting phosphorous derivatives.

2 Why is this important?

The World Health Organization (WHO) cites globalization, consumerism, growth in free markets, increased cross-border communication and the ubiquity of the Internet as agents of change in medicine and pharmaceuticals, giving rise to new safety concerns. Furthermore, the increasingly global trade in pharmaceuticals and higher levels of regulatory complexity have impelled many intergovernmental organisations to make efforts towards harmonisation of regulatory activities to ensure consistent efficacy of pharmacovigilance efforts (WHO 2002).

Medication errors make up a high proportion of all patient safety events (Jordan & Kyriacos 2014; Ostini *et al.* 2012) and some result in overdose or adverse drug reactions, and can cause serious harm to patients (Aronson 2009); Runciman *et al.* 2003). Medication incidents in the UK resulted in 50 deaths between October 2011 and September 2012 (Jordan & Kyriacos 2014). It is estimated that medication errors cost the USA between $15bn and $28bn each year and that the USA spent an additional $213bn (8% of total healthcare spend) in 2012 on costs arising from medicines mismanagement, including medication errors (Aitken & Valkova 2013).

Medication errors may be a result of medicines having names that look alike or sound alike and are referred to as *LASA errors*. Examples of confused LASA pairs are given in (2).

(2) a. *mercaptamine-mercaptopurine.* A 9-month-old infant presented with nephropathic cystinosis and was prescribed mercaptopurine by the GP instead of mercaptamine. After a month on the wrong medication, she developed pancytopenia but ultimately made a full recovery (MHPRA 2010).

b. *hydromorphone-morphine.* An elderly patient was discharged after being administered hydromorphone instead of the prescribed morphine by a nurse in the Emergency Department. He suffered a fatal respiratory arrest on his way home.

LASA errors are estimated to account for around 25% of all medication errors in the US (Emmerton & Rizk 2012), and occur in all aspects of medications management – during prescribing, dispensing and administration of the medication. LASA errors thus represent a significant threat to patient safety.

The bulk of extant literature on LASA errors focuses on mitigating their occurrence (Emmerton & Rizk 2012; Ghaleb *et al.* 2010, Aronson 2009; Kovacic & Chambers 2011) and very little research has been conducted into linguistic properties of the nomenclature to elucidate properties that may prime the risk of the errors occurring. Profiling of such properties could inform the name formation process and thus prophylactically reduce the risk to patient safety. It is also possible that elucidating external factors contributing to the likelihood of confusion error (such as high syllabic similarity) will encourage reporting of adverse drug events (ADEs) and near misses, since these may be under-reported due in part to fear of reprisal, blame and reputation damage (Aronson 2009).

More needs to be known about the formal and semantic properties of the main global medication nomenclature of International Nonproprietary Names. This study examines semantic transparency in the nomenclature and the underlying conceptual taxonomy of pharmacological relationship. In the context of this study, semantic transparency is defined as the correspondence between form and meaning within a lexical unit and the extent to which meaning motivates form and meaning is derived from form.

3 Medical taxonomies and ontologies

There are many systems of classification in medicine, such as the HUGO (HUman Genome Organisation) gene nomenclature, Medical Subject Headings (MeSH) used to index published research on Medline, and the University of Washington Digital Anatomist (UWDA) (Shapiro *et al.* 2005; Segura-Bedmar *et al.* 2008). Due to the exponential growth of published research in medicine, it is now impossible for specialists to keep abreast of developments in their field, and the need has arisen to automate recognition of key concepts in the literature (Coletti & Bleich 2001, Segura-Bedmar *et al.* 2008). The Unified Medical Language System (UMLS) is an example of an ontology by which automated software can read and assimilate information in published research (Segura-Bedmar *et al.* 2008) and encompasses various nodes, such as the UWDA for anatomy. Some systems determine nomenclature, such as the HUGO gene nomenclature, and others are used to assign conceptual relations, such as the UWDA (Shapiro *et al.* 2005). The UWDA uses various semantic links, e.g. the oesophagus is *part-of* the foregut, *continuous-with* the pharynx and stomach and *adjacent-to* the trachea, thoracic aorta and thoracic vertebral column.

The terms *classification*, *taxonomy* and *ontology* are often used interchangeably to refer to any system of categorization, but for the purposes of this study, *ontology* is taken to mean any system that categorizes concepts (Stevens *et al.* 2000) and a taxonomy should be seen as a methodology for categorization. There are several key distinctions to be made. An ontology is "the concrete form of a conceptualization of a community's knowledge of a domain" (2000: 1), whereas a taxonomy does not necessarily include added knowledge beyond the necessary and sufficient criteria for categorization. Ontologies may be multidirectional and include multiple types of semantic relation, such as meronymy and metonymy, whereas a taxonomy is an upside down tree structure (Shapiro *et al.* 2005) and is based upon intrinsic properties of its members. Taxonomies are typically 'tree-like' hierarchies, employing hyponymy (*is-a*, class membership) to express semantic relationship. In terms of Jackendoff's widely adopted theory, the organization of systems will inevitably depend upon our conceptualization of the world (Jackendoff 1983), but further consideration of that is beyond the scope of this chapter. The prototypical taxonomy is the plant or animal kingdom used in biology (Shapiro *et al.* 2005, Coletti & Bleich 2001).

According to the WHO, the INN system is a 'classification', but can be more specifically defined as a taxonomy since it only employs *is-a*, hyponymic semantic relations. Although there is a global taxonomic system for pharmaceutical substances, the Anatomical Therapeutic Chemical (ATC) index, INNs use a different taxonomy that does not align with the ATC (Segura-Bedmar *et al.* 2008) and is not used by any other organization. For example, the medication name *selegiline* in the ATC system would be found by drilling down into the taxonomy: Nervous system > Anti-parkinson drugs > Dopaminergic agents > Monoamine oxidase B inhibitors, but in the INN system by Psychopharmacologics > Antidepressants > Monoamine oxidase inhibitors.

The INN system employs at most a four-level taxonomy and assigns alphanumeric codes to each level. Although there is room for four levels, currently names fill only two levels, so the INN system can be seen as a flat taxonomy or a collection of individual taxa under an undefined hyperonym. There is sparse information on the taxonomy beyond the statutory guidance of the WHO and neither definitions nor necessary and sufficient criteria for inclusion in the taxonomy are provided. The INN system is unique in the world of medical ontologies and taxonomies in that the nomenclature it motivates is used by people at all levels of society who hold varying levels of knowledge.

4 A typology of taxa in the INN nomenclature

Pharmacological relationships between substances are demonstrated by the use of a common stem (WHO 1997: 1), which may be a prefix, infix, suffix, or a 'freefix'. By using a common stem, the INN indicates that its denoted substance belongs to a group of substances with similar pharmacological activity (WHO 1997: 1). The common stem or sub-stem is combined with a "random, fantasy prefix", normally chosen by the submitter of the new substance (WHO 1997: 6) and "the only requirement is to contribute to a euphonious and distinctive name" (WHO 2004: 128). Displaying taxonomy from right to left, starting at the end of the name, is a predictable approach for the user as they can first categorize the name under its stem and further sub-categorize under sub-stems by reading to the left. The reverse would be impossible due to the meaningless prefix. The INN taxonomy is based upon hyponymy, and in this chapter, *stem* will be used to denote hyperonym and *sub-stem* to denote hyponym.

This chapter presents a qualitative typology of taxa found in the INN nomenclature and reviews the implications of these types in the usability of INNs. WHO guidance stipulates that names must not be liable to confusion and that relationship must be shown by the use of a common stem. Therefore, there must be a robust and structured underlying conceptual taxonomy in place to facilitate correct usage of the medication names. The typology that follows is a qualitative analysis of the author's database of monolexic INNs (n=7,111) and the *WHO Stem Book* 2011, which provides information on the INN taxonomy and lists of INNs containing each stem and sub-stem (WHO 2011).

4.1 Single-level taxa

There are many INNs that are regularly formed, some with only a single-level taxon represented by a single stem. This type of taxon has no hyponyms. Examples are given in Table 1-1 overleaf. These stems occur as all four types of affix: prefix, infix, suffix and freefix.

These single-level taxa illustrate the longevity of the INN nomenclature: from its inception in 1952, the taxonomy has allowed for developments in pharmacology by creating empty pharmacological taxa. Stems are created, but may not appear in names immediately – the system is proactive rather than reactive. This future-proofing is similar to Dmitri Mendeleev's periodic table, in which gaps were left for elements not yet discovered. It is possible that in future a sub-category of cannabinoid receptor agonists may be discovered and in that case a sub-stem of *nab* can be created.

Stem	*Affix type*	*Pharmacology*	*Examples of INNs*
arte-	prefix	antimalarial agents, artemisinin related compounds	arteflene, arterolane
-coxib	suffix	selective cyclo-oxygenase inhibitors	etoricoxib, tilmacoxib
-formin	suffix	antihyperglycaemics, phenformin derivatives	benfosformin, metformin
nab	freefix	cannabinoid receptor agonists	menabitan, nonabine
-pris-	infix	steroidal compounds acting on progesterone receptors	ulipristal, asoprisnil

Table 1-1: Examples of single-level taxa[2]

4.2 Regular taxa

Many stem taxa clearly display their taxonomy in names that can be interpreted from right to left. The stem is the suffix and sub-stems are distinguished from their co-hyponyms as infixes directly before the suffix stem. The taxon for "antiasthmatic, antiallergic substances not acting primarily as antihistaminics" has the stem *-ast*, and sub-stems *-lukast*, *-milast*, *-trodast* and *-zolast*. Montelukast is a substance in this group and its meaning can be easily derived from the order of word parts: the suffix stem *-ast* can be used to categorize the substance as part of the antiasthmatic taxon and the infix *-luk-* can be used to further sub-categorize it as a leukotriene receptor antagonist.

In regular taxa such as these, morphemic concatenation is ordered as in Table 1-2.

[2] The hyphen indicates the position of the affix in the name. Freefixes are unhyphenated to indicate they can appear in any position.

Random prefix	***Sub-stem (distinguishing part)***	***Stem***	***INN***
andol		ast	andolast
monte	luk	ast	montelukast
teto	mil	ast	tetomilast
sero	trod	ast	serotrodast
qua	zol	ast	quazolast

Table 1-2: Morphemic concatenation in the *-ast* stem taxon

4.3 Monoclonal antibodies: a complex and regular taxon

Monoclonal antibodies are a relatively new but rapidly growing branch of biochemistry and their INN taxon is complex but well defined. There is a regular correspondence between names in this group and their meaning, and meaning is predictable for the user. INNs for monoclonal antibodies comprise a random prefix, followed by two infixes referring to, respectively, the target organ or disease of the medication and the source species on which the immunoglobulin sequence is based, and the hyperonymic stem *-mab*.

Each of the three meaning-bearing elements must be defined in the name and concatenated in a certain order, but they combine freely with each other.

In this complex and regular taxon, morphemic concatenation is ordered as in Table 1-3.

Ran-dom prefix	***Sub-stem 1 (target)***	***Sub-stem 2 (source)***	***Stem***	***INN***	***Description***
icru	c	u	mab	icrucumab	targeting cardiovascul-ar system, of human origin
siru	k	u	mab	sirukumab	targeting interleukin, of human origin
ce	tu	xi	mab	cetuximab	targeting tumours, of chimeric origin
ur	toxa	zu	mab	urtoxa-zumab	targeting toxin, of humanized origin

Table 1-3: Morphemic concatenation in the *-mab* stem taxon

The complete *-mab* taxon is shown in Table 1-4.

sub-stem 1 - target	***sub-stem 2 - source***	***stem***	
		-mab	monoclonal antibody
	-a-		rat
	-axo-		rat/mouse
	-e-		hamster
	-i-		primate
	-o-		mouse
	-u-		human
	-xi-		chimeric
	-xizu-		chimeric/ humanised
	-zu-		humanised
-b(a)-			bacterial
-c(i)-			cardiovascular
-f(u)-			fungal
-k(i)-			interleukin
-l(i)-			immunomodulating
-n(e)-			neural
-s(o)-			bone
-tox(a)-			toxin

Table 1-4 *-mab* stem taxon

There are eight infixes to denote the target class and nine infixes to denote the source class, although not all of these are currently used in INNs. These may be combined freely with each other but the order in which they appear in the name is fixed. As an example, *urtoxazumab*, which refers to a humanized monoclonal antibody directed against a type of toxin-producing Escherichia Coli (E. Coli), can be decomposed as *ur-toxa-zu-mab*, in which *-toxa-* indicates that it targets a toxin, and *-zu-* indicates that it is humanized (derived from a non-human antibody, which has been engineered to be more homologous with human antibodies). This is not an example of a three-tiered taxonomy, but rather two mutually independent parameters of classification under a single hyperonym.

Infixes have two forms depending on the following letter; for example, *-tox(a)-* is realized as *-toxa-* in the above example because it is followed by a consonant. In *actoxumab*, it is realized as *-tox-* because it is followed by the vocalic infix *-u-*. Without optional linking elements, INNs may contain phonemes outside the phonotactics of English (such as **urtoxzumab*) and thus run the risk of being mispronounced and misunderstood. In names for monoclonal antibodies, meaning is conveyed in almost every component of the word and even in a single letter, thus optimizing the space available and minimizing character redundancy.

4.4 Irregular display of taxonomy

For names within some taxa, there are very clear concatenation rules for stems and sub-stems. For example, in names for monoclonal antibodies the distinguishing part of the hyponym is prefixed to the stem of its hyperonym in the name. However, often the formation of sub-stems for hyponyms of a main stem is not consistent in INNs, given the variation in types of affix used. The taxon for antivirals with the stem *vir* will be used as an example. As a freefix, the stem *vir* can appear anywhere in the name, meaning that the user cannot rely on a right-to-left display of taxonomy to derive the meaning. The stem has sub-stems *-amivir, -asvir, -buvir, -anvir, -buvir -cavir, -ciclovir, -fovir, -gosivir, -navir, -previr, -virine* and *-viroc*.

In irregular taxa such as these, there are two orders of morphemic concatenation, exemplified in (3).

(3) a. alamifovir (random prefix: *alami*; distinguishing part of sub-stem: *-fo-*; stem: *vir*)
b. vicriviroc (random prefix: *vicri*; stem: *vir*; distinguishing part of sub-stem: *-oc*)

The meaning of *alamifovir* in (3a) can easily be derived from the order of morphemic concatenation in the name. However, in *vicriviroc* in (3b), the distinguishing part of the hyponymic sub-stem *-viroc* follows its hyperonym in the name and thus it is not immediately obvious to which taxon the name belongs. A user may mistakenly categorize the name under the stem **-oc*, which does not exist. This can also be seen in other stem taxa, such as the hyperonym *prost* with hyponym *-prostil*, and in any taxon for which the stem is not a suffix. This problem arises from the phenomenon of freefixes in INNs. As freefix stems such as *vir* and *prost* do not have a set position in the name, semantic transparency may be low since the user has no predictable way of recognizing the main stem.

4.5 Morphosemantics

As is clear from regular stem taxa and the monoclonal antibodies taxon, morphemic order is important for the easy recognition of INNs. When stems are suffixes and sub-stems are infixes, taxonomy is displayed and semantic transparency is high.

In some stem taxa, meaning is motivated solely by morphemic order: sub-stems take the same form as the stem and are distinguishable only by their position in the name. The *-fos* stem taxon denoting "insecticides, anthelminthics, pesticides etc, phosphorous derivatives" will be used as an example. When *-fos* is used as a suffix, it is the hyperonym of the taxon. When it appears as an infix or a prefix, it is the hyponym denoting "various pharmacological categories belonging to fos, other than those above" (an insufficient differentiation, but nonetheless confirming its hyponym status). This messy taxon may be mistaken for a single category with a freefix stem, but in fact the position of the stem in the name motivates meaning.

Freefixes disturb semantic transparency in INNs by creating unpredictability in morphemic order and they cause inconsistency. Users must learn that in some cases meaning depends on the position of the stem in the name and that in other cases position does not matter.

4.6 Allomorphy

A stem may have several orthographic allomorphs, illustrated by the examples in Table 1-5. These are variant forms of the stem that do not indicate a change in meaning. Allomorphy in this sense can be dangerous: when pharmacological relationship is differentiated in units as small as a single letter, allomorphs such as *-profen* and *-profene* may lead to confusion in other areas. For example, *-fenin* and *-fenine* are separate stem families denoting "diagnostic aids; (phenylcarbamoyl)methyl iminodiacetic acid derivatives" and "analgesics, glafenine derivatives", respectively, but are only distinguished by a final letter *-e*. Variation in the orthographic form of stems under a common hyperonym can obfuscate meaning and may also falsely suggest a relationship where there is none.

Official stem	*Examples*	*Allo-morphs*	*Examples*
-azepam (diazepam derivatives)	diazepam, lorazepam	-azam;	arfendazam, clobazam
-cillin (antibiotics, 6-aminopenicillanic acid derivatives)	penicillin, amoxicillin	-cillide; -cillinam	libecillide; bacmecillinam, pivmecillinam
-eridine (analgesics, pethidine derivatives)	morpheridine, properidine	-ethidine	pethidine, [3] hydroxy-pethidine
-izine (diphenylmethyl piperazine derivatives)	cetirizine, cyclizine	-yzine	hydroxyzine
-mantadine (adamantane derivatives)	amantadine, somantadine	-mantine; -mantone	memantine, dopamantine; idramantone
-profen (anti-inflammatory agents, ibuprofen derivatives)	ibuprofen, tetriprofen	-profene	aprofene, diprofene
-tril (endopeptidase inhibitors)	dexecadotril, candoxatril	-trilat	omepatrilat, sampatrilat

Table 1-5: Allomorphy

5 Discussion

As Saussure highlighted with his analogy of the linguistic sign and the two sides of a piece of paper (Sanders 2004), the formal and semantic aspects of language are inextricably linked; formal aspects of INNs are motivated by their underlying semantics and although the formal realization of INNs may be conducive to conveying meaning, it can equally misrepresent

[3] The example of *pethidine* highlights the difference between the accepted linguistic use of *stem* and the use of this term in the context of INNs. In *pethidine*, *-ethidine* is the stem, and *p-* is the random prefix assigned to distinguish it from others in its stem family.

meaning and increase the risk of confusion. Although meaning is primarily derived through the taxonomic system, it is also motivated by the class of affix and the ordering within the name of stems and sub-stems.

The pharmaceutical nomenclature and its peripheral systems of nomenclature are large and complex. A taxonomic conceptual system developed over a number of decades will inevitably contain some broken links and general inconsistencies, but these inconsistencies should not work to the detriment of the overall aim of the system. The structure of the INN taxonomy does not conform to the archetypal tree structure and is at times messy and fractured. Properly structured taxonomies help to bring substantial order to a model, whereas improperly structured taxonomies make models confusing and difficult to use (Guarino & Welty 2000). A robust taxonomy is also important for automated recognition systems and this will increase the life-span and usage of the INN nomenclature (Segura-Bedmar *et al.* 2008).

Semantic motivation in International Nonproprietary Names is multifaceted, encompassing multiple methods of conveying meaning. The INN nomenclature does not sufficiently exploit formal aspects of language by using a systematic and linear ordering of stems and sub-stems in the name, thus resulting in pharmacologically related sub-stems that appear to be unrelated, such as *-ciclovir* and *-viroc*. This type of hyponymy defeats the object of a nomenclature to reflect a deep classification of concepts, as the formal realization gives no indication of its paradigmatic relations. Of course, there are many instances of nested concepts that are mirrored in the formal realization, such as the naming of monoclonal antibodies with the stem *-mab* and two systems of infix sub-stems and the designation of single stems that do belong to a taxon of related stems does not present too many problems.

There is no single way for a user to predict meaning, and the burden of learning on clinical users (pharmacists, nurses, physicians, medical students) is high. They must understand not only the meanings of stems and the layout of the taxonomy, but also the inconsistencies peculiar to each stem taxon. They need to know that meaning may be motivated at the morphemic level by the class of affix and the morphemic concatenation of stems and sub-stems and to know when to ignore spelling variation and when to take note of a single letter bearing meaning. It is little wonder that in practice, clinicians rely instead on the gradual learning of whole names and memorize them based upon their spelling and phonology (personal communication with Dr. Sue Jordan, Swansea University). Many stem taxa, such as those for monoclonal antibodies, are complex but regular and there is a predictable display of taxonomy and correspondence between form and meaning. Semantic transparency in many of the resulting names is low and marred by inconsistency.

The exact interplay between transparency and similarity is currently unclear, since my preliminary observations suggest that in some cases, transparency will increase orthographic similarity between names and thus increase the risk of confusion, yet without transparency, users would need to learn thousands of names by rote. Given the risk to patient safety in this rapidly expanding field, the system of international pharmaceutical nomenclature certainly warrants further linguistic investigation.

6 Conclusion

INNs carry out different functions depending on the user, and thus they must be understandable at multiple levels. For patients and non-professionals they must be recognizable and pronounceable, but at the same time, they must 'whisper' in the ear of health professionals by communicating meaning through neoclassical compounds and the general norms of pharmaceutical nomenclature. To facilitate the correct realization of each INN in all four modalities of language (listening, reading, speaking and writing) and thus to prevent confusion between INNs, it is imperative that formal aspects are controlled and fully optimized.

The WHO has been described as the "locus of efforts to improve global health … which is the foundation for peace and prosperity" (Council for Foreign Relations 2012). Global stewardship is an essential role of the WHO in how it identifies needs to be met and takes a leadership role in setting global norms (Clark *et al.* 2010). Given the primary objective of the WHO, "the attainment by all peoples of the highest possible level of health", the INN programme must always be viewed from the perspective of patient safety. By creating an international nomenclature that is publicly available worldwide, it acts as a fulcrum between various institutions operating within separate strata of the pharmaceutical industry and inevitably paves the way for more global consistency and communication, ultimately enhancing the safety of patients.

References

Aitken, Murray & Valkova, Silvia (2013), *Avoidable Costs in U.S. Healthcare*, Parsippany (NJ): IMS Institute for Healthcare Informatics.
Aronson, Jeffrey K. (2000), 'Where name and image meet – the argument for adrenaline', *BMJ* 320(7233): 506-509.

—. (2009), 'Medication errors: what they are, how they happen, and how to avoid them', *QJM: Monthly Journal of the Association of Physicians* 102(8): 513-521.

Clark, William C.; Szlezak, Nicole A.; Moon, Suerie; Bloom, Barry R.; Keusch, Gerald T.; Michaud, Catherine M.; Jamison, Dean T.; Frenk, Julio & Kilama Wen L. (2010), 'The Global Health System: Institutions in a Time of Transition. Harvard University, Centre for International Development: Working Paper 193', http://www.hks.harvard.edu/var/ezp_site/storage/fckeditor/image/center-programs/cid/publications/193.pdf (viewed 19 Nov. 2014).

Council on Foreign Relations (CFR) (2012), 'Global Governance Monitor: Public Health', http://www.cfr.org/global-governance/global-governance-monitor/p18985?breadcrumb=%2Fthinktank%2Fiigg%2Fpublications#/Public%20Health/Overview%20Video (viewed 1 Oct. 2014).

Coletti, Margaret H. & Bleich, Howard L. (2001), 'Medical Subject Headings Used to Search the Biomedical Literature', *Journal of the American Medical Informatics Association* 8(4): 317-323.

Deléger, Louise; Namer, Fiammetta & Zweigenbaum, Pierre (2009), 'Morphosemantic parsing of medical compound words: transferring a French analyzer to English', *International Journal of Medical Informatics* 78(1): 48-55.

Emmerton, Lynne M. & Rizk, Mariam F. S. (2012), 'Look-alike and sound-alike medicines: risks and "solutions"', *International Journal of Clinical Pharmacy* 34(1): 4-8.

Ghaleb, Maisoon A.; Barber, Nick; Franklin, Bryony D. & Wong, Ian C. K. (2010), 'The incidence and nature of prescribing and medication administration errors in paediatric inpatients', *Archives of Disease in Childhood* 95(2): 113-118.

Guarino, Nicola & Welty, Christopher (2000), 'Ontological Analysis of Taxonomic Relationships', in Juris Hartmanis & van Leeuwen, Jan (eds.), *Lecture notes in computer science*, Germany: Max-Planck Institute of Computer Science, 210-224.

Institute for Safe Medication Practices (ISMP) (2011), 'List of confused drug names', http://www.ismp.org/tools/confuseddrugnames.pdf (viewed 3 Oct. 2014).

Jackendoff, Ray S. (1983), *Semantics and Cognition*, London: MIT.

Jordan, Sue & Kyriacos, Una (2014), 'Medicines' management: a public health problem on nursing's agenda', *Journal of Nursing Management* 22(3): 271-275.

Kovacic, Laurel & Chambers, Carole (2011), 'Look-alike, sound-alike drugs in oncology', *Journal of Oncology Pharmacy Practice* 17(2): 104-118.

Marecková, Elena; Simon, Frantisek & Cerveny, Ladislav (2002), 'Latin as the language of medical terminology: some remarks on its role and prospects', *Swiss Medical Weekly* 23: 581-587.

Medicines and Healthcare Products Regulatory Agency (MHPRA) (2010), 'Mercaptamine and mercaptopurine: confusion between drug names', https://www.gov.uk/drug-safety-update/mercaptamine-and-mercaptopurine-confusion-between-drug-names (viewed 18 Feb. 2015).

Ostini, Remo; Roughead, Elizabeth E.; Kirkpatrick, Carl M. J.; Monteith, Greg R. & Tett, Susan E. (2012), 'Quality Use of Medicines-medication safety issues in naming; look-alike, sound-alike medicine names', *International Journal of Pharmacy Practice*, 20(6): 349-357.

Runciman, William B.; Roughead, Elizabeth E.; Semple, Susan J. & Adams, Robert J. (2003), 'Adverse drug events and medication errors in Australia', *International Journal for Quality in Health Care* 15(90001): 49-59.

Sanders, Carole (2004), *The Cambridge Companion to Saussure*, Cambridge: Cambridge University Press.

Segura-Bedmar, Isabel; Martínez, Paloma & Segura-Bedmar, María (2008), 'Drug name recognition and classification in biomedical texts. A case study outlining approaches underpinning automated systems', *Drug Discovery Today* 13(17-18): 816-823.

Shapiro, Linda G.; Chung, Emily; Detwiler, Landon T.; Mejino, José L. V.; Agoncillo, Augusto V; Brinkley, James F. & Rosse, Cornelius (2005), 'Processes and problems in the formative evaluation of an interface to the Foundational Model of Anatomy knowledge base', *Journal of the American Medical Informatics Association (JAMIA)* 12(1): 35-46.

Stevens, Robert; Goble, Carole A. & Bechhofer, Sean (2000), 'Ontology-based knowledge representation for bioinformatics', *Briefings in bioinformatics* 1(4): 398-414.

World Health Organization (WHO) (1997), 'Guidance on the Use of International Nonproprietary Names (INNs) for Pharmaceutical Substances', http://whqlibdoc.who.int/hq/1997/who_pharm_s_nom_1570.pdf (viewed 21 Oct. 2014).

WHO (2002), 'The importance of pharmacovigilance', http://whqlibdoc.who.int/hq/2002/a75646.pdf (viewed 21 Oct. 2014).

—. (2004), 'The use of stems in the selection of International Nonproprietary Names (INN) for pharmaceutical substances', http://whqlibdoc.who.int/hq/2004/WHO_EDM_QSM_2004.5.pdf (viewed 27 Oct. 11).
—. (2011), 'WHO StemBook 2011: The use of stems in the selection of International Nonproprietary Names (INN) for pharmaceutical substances', http://www.who.int/medicines/services/inn/StemBook_2011_Final.pdf (viewed 3 Feb. 2014).

CHAPTER TWO

TERM VARIATION IN THE PSYCHIATRIC DOMAIN: TRANSPARENCY AND MULTIDIMENSIONALITY

PILAR LEÓN-ARAÚZ

Medicine is one of the most dynamic terminological domains, since knowledge is constantly evolving and many different user types and situations are involved in medical communication. This dynamism usually causes a great deal of term variation for several reasons and with diverse consequences. The choice of one term or the other depends on different communicative and cognitive factors. For instance, in a doctor-patient situation, the doctor will often address the patient with rather transparent terms, whereas in a medical conference they will use the most standardized form. On the other hand, the terms designating medical concepts may change and evolve as new discoveries are made or as negative connotations arise. For example, it was only after discovering that *Down syndrome* was caused by the presence of an extra chromosome that the variant *trisomy 21* emerged, focusing on the causal dimension of the concept. Until then, the variants designating such a concept focused on the discoverer of the disease (John Langdon Down, 1828-1896) or the physical attributes of the patients (*mongolism*), which would finally be suppressed due to (obvious) negative connotations. Thus, the representation of term variants is a key component of any terminological resource which addresses translators. This is the main aim of the research project VariMed (varimed.ugr.es), a multifunctional resource on the medical domain for linguistic research, translation and technical writing (Tercedor Sánchez et al. 2014).

In this paper, I show how different naming devices emerge in the field of psychiatry and how we classify them in VariMed according to different parameters. As stated by Candel Mora and Carrió Pastor (2012), discovering the causes or types of variation is important for both theoretical and practical reasons. From a theoretical perspective, it may reflect the mental processes involved in the selection of one term over the other. On a practical level, it could be helpful to terminologists or translators in production tasks, since they need to know when and why to select one particular variant over the rest. In this sense, Rogers (1997) underlines that translators must regularly make decisions not only concerning synonymy within the source text and within the target text, but also concerning the cross-linguistic relations between these synonyms. Our aim is to discover the motivations behind the use of the different variants in terms of communicative and cognitive parameters. In this chapter, communicative parameters are understood in terms of the expert-lay continuum (e.g. the knowledge shared by text senders and receivers), whereas cognitive parameters are based on the different conceptual dimensions activated by the choice of each term (multidimensionality) and its collocational context. This chapter is structured as follows. In Section 1, I give a brief overview on term variation and multidimensionality. In Section 2, the representation of term variants in VariMed is explained. In Section 3, I analyse the correlation among different factors underlying term variation in a 10 million-word corpus on psychiatry, in particular (1) conceptual dimensions and text types, (2) term variants and text types, and (3) term variants and collocational context. Finally, I draw some conclusions in Section 5.

1 Transparency and multidimensionality in term variation

Although specialized language was initially intended to have one linguistic designation for each concept for greater precision, it is true that the same concept can often have many different types of linguistic designations. At first sight, the use of one variant or the other might seem arbitrary. However, Rogers (1997:219) shows that there are certain systematic patterns of variation that need to be explained. In the same line, Bowker and Hawkins (2006) do not believe that variation can be attributed to carelessness on the part of the subject field experts, but rather that experts formulate their expressions carefully to ensure that the information transmitted is as precise as possible.

In the same way as in general language, there is terminological variation influenced by user-based parameters of geographic, temporal or social variation or usage-based parameters of tenor, field and mode (Gregory and Carroll 1978). Nevertheless, terminological variation also occurs for reasons that are often considerably more complex and difficult to explain. Freixa (2006: 52) classifies the causes for terminological variation in the following categories: (1) dialectal, caused by different origins of the authors; (2) functional, caused by different communicative registers; (3) discursive, caused by different stylistic and expressive needs of the authors; (4) interlinguistic, caused by contact between languages; (5) cognitive, caused by different conceptualizations and motivations. According to Freixa (2002), cognitive term variants are not only formally different, but also semantically diverse, as they give a particular vision of the concept. In this sense, Fernández-Silva (2010) and Fernández-Silva et al. (2011) describe this phenomenon as the linguistic reflection of conceptual multidimensionality, whereas Bowker (1998) points to multidimensionality as one of the potential causes for the apparent randomness of term choice.

Multidimensionality has been defined by many authors (Bowker 1997, Kageura 1997, Wright 1997, Rogers 2004) as the phenomenon in which certain concepts can be classified according to different points of view or conceptual facets. This has important consequences for how domains are categorized and modelled (León-Araúzet al. 2013). According to Picht and Draskau (1985, 48 quoted by Rogers 2004: 219), multidimensionality depends on who is the classifier as well as the different knowledge sources that may reflect different criteria when organizing the same domain or knowledge node. For example, botanists would classify roses differently from rose growers. However, multidimensionality has also an impact on term variation, since a concept can be designated in more than one way based on the different characteristics that it possesses (Fernández-Silva et al. 2014). Thus, term variation should not be regarded as a linguistic phenomenon isolated from conceptual representations, since the choice of one term instead of another is the result of different perspectives towards reality.

In our study, we have found many different types of term variants for the same concept. Some of them were just acronyms, dialectal, orthographic or morphological variants, which, of course, need to be stored in any terminological resource (see Section 3), but in this chapter I focus especially on dimensional variant types, which need more in-depth study, since they affect both cognitive and communicative situations. Dimensional variants show different conceptualizations of the same concept according to different facets or dimensions. For instance, *Ganser syndrome*, *nonsense syndrome* and *prison psychosis* are all variants of the same concept, but the first one highlights a discoverer dimension (Sigbert Ganser, 1853-1931, was the first to describe the syndrome), the second one focuses on the symptom dimension (saying nonsense is one of them) and the third one on the location dimension (it often takes place in prisons, since it affects inmates).

In terminological resources, users are often confronted with a vast array of variants with no other information on how term variation arises and how their use may be constrained. Nevertheless, they need to know when to use each of the variants and the conceptual connotations they imply, since this will affect the receiver's interpretation of the message. Otherwise, translators may actually over-standardize, where the use of variants was deliberate and well-reasoned (Bowker and Hawkins, 2006: 80), because translators often tend to ignore terminological variation for the sake of consistency (Merkel, 1996).

Dimensional variant types are codified in compound nouns that are usually transparent multi-word terms (e.g. A+N: *affective disorder*; A+A+N: *acute delusional disorder*; A+N+N: *acute stress disorder*; N+N+N: *hair pulling disorder*), although single-word compound terms can also be found (e.g. *bedwetting*). According to Bowker (1998), compounding achieves two objectives. It narrows a concept's intention, thereby creating a closer determination of the concept, and at the same time, it shows the relation that exists between the new concept and its origin. Thus, compounding often reflects a higher degree of transparency than terms resulting from other naming devices.

Transparency is often understood as the easiness with which anyone can understand the meaning of the term by inferring it from the meaning of its constituents. However, in terminology very technical constituents can also make a compound noun more opaque, even if the meaning of the term is the combination of each constituent's meaning. For instance, *enuresis* and *bedwetting* designate the same concept and are formed through the same naming device: different morphemes forming a single-word term. *Enuresis* has a Greek origin and is constituted by the morphemes *en* (on) + *ur* (urinate) + *esis* (condition). It reveals a pattern in transparent term formation from an etymological point of view, but not for lay receivers, who would more easily understand the *bedwetting* choice. Therefore, compounding, transparency and dimensional variants are intimately linked in an expert-lay continuum that should be further analysed based on corpus evidence.

2 Representing term variants in VariMed

In the terminological knowledge base of VariMed, concepts and terms are represented according to different descriptive fields. In Figure 2-1, the concept GANSER SYNDROME is represented through a definition, its related concepts (in this case, hyperonyms), the organ affected (brain) and all of its term variants. Concept entries are often accompanied by illustrative images, but in the case of psychiatric concepts, images are less useful and thus less frequent.

concepto*	SÍNDROME DE GANSER - GANSER SYNDROME
definición*	trastorno facticio en el que el individuo se caracteriza por responder a las preguntas de una manera aproximada, sin sentido o evidentemente errónea.
tipo*	enfermedad
conceptos asociados	• SÍNDROME DE GANSER tipo de **TRASTORNO DISOCIATIVO** • SÍNDROME DE GANSER tipo de **TRASTORNO FACTICIO**
órganos	• cerebro
imágenes	
variantes	• **balderdash syndrome** (en) • **Ganser syndrome** (en) • **nonsense syndrome** (en) • **prison psychosis** (en) • **pseudodemencia histérica** (es) • **psicosis carcelaria** (es) • **síndrome de Ganser** (es) • **syndrome of approximate answers** (es)

Fig. 2-1: Concept entry of GANSER SYNDROME in VariMed

Variants also have their own term entry, as shown in Figure 2-2.

variante*	Ganser syndrome
concepto*	**SÍNDROME DE GANSER** enfermedad
categoría gramatical	unidad fraseológica
idioma*	en
registro*	formal
otra marca	• epónimo
dimensiones	• investigador-descubridor

Fig. 2-2: Term entry of *Ganser syndrome* in VariMed

They are related to the concept they designate and to other different fields, such as language, part of speech, register, conceptual dimensions and other features.

Some of these other features are linked to the different naming devices involved in term formation (borrowings, calques, eponyms, acronyms, etc.), as depicted in Table 2-1. But they also include other usage-related information, such as the fields ICD-10 (International Classification of Diseases) and MeSH (Medical Subject Headings), which show standardized forms; or deprecated and obsolete, which discourage the use of certain terms.

Data category	***Descriptive field value***	***Example***
Register	Formal	*bruxism*
	Informal	*teeth clenching*
	Experts-informal	*punch-drunk syndrome*
	Neutral	*panic attack*
	Children	*belly pain*
	Affects_population	*infantile autism*
	Cause	*alcohol-induced amnestic disorder*

Dimensions	Attribute	*psychogenic fugue*
	Composed_of	*nodular melanoma*
	Time	*seasonal affective disorder*
	Intensity	*mild cognitive impairment*
	Discoverer	*Cotard delusion*
	Body_part	*wet brain*
	Metaphor/metonymy	*Fred Astaire legs*
	Location	*prison psychosis*
Other features	Ortographic variant	*nonfluent aphasia*
	Shortening	*flu*
	English calque	*afasia no fluente* (Spanish)
	French calque	*locura a dos* (Spanish)
	Eponym	*Alzheimer's disease*
	False friend	*trauma*
	Misspelling	*gall stone*
	Neologism	*niebla mental*
	ICD-10	*Wernicke's encephalopathy*
	MeSH	*anorexia nervosa*
	Greek or Latin origin	*chorea sacti viti*
	English borrowing	*síndrome de burnout*
	Borrowing from other languages	*bouffée délirante*
	Acronym	*BMS (burning mouth syndrome)*
	Cultural term	*amok*
	Deprecated term	*mental retardation*
	Obsolete term	*depressive personality*

Table 2-1: Descriptive fields of term entries in VariMed

Most examples in Table 2-1 are drawn from the psychiatric domain, but some of them are not because there are certain features that do not apply in this domain. For instance, children are not usually familiarized with psychiatric disorders. Thus, no children-type register has been found in the domain yet. Since VariMed has a multi-functional purpose, which means that even doctors could use it in multilingual doctor-patient situations, the children register has also been included in order to conduct familiarity studies across different settings. In the same way, the experts-informal register has been introduced in order to distinguish the informal jargon used by doctors from the colloquialisms used by patients.

The register fields are mutually exclusive, but the conceptual dimensions and other features can coexist. For example, BMS is an acronym (*burning mouth syndrome*) and at the same time it shows two dimensions: Body_part and Symptom. Cultural terms and metaphors are usually intimately related. For example, terms such as *Münchhausen syndrome*, *Alice in Wonderland syndrome*, *Lilliputian hallucinations* or *knight's move thinking* are formed through culture-based metaphorical extensions according to the patient's symptoms. The first syndrome, which is a factitious disorder, enhances the symptom dimension by referring to Baron Münchhausen, a popular fictional character that tells fantastic stories about himself. Focusing on the same dimension, there are other, more transparent variants for this syndrome, such as *hospital addiction syndrome, hospital hopper syndrome*, and other metaphorical variants, such as *thick chart syndrome. Alice in Wonderland syndrome* and *Lilliputian hallucinations* are both term variants for the same concept: MICROPSIA, a condition in which objects are perceived smaller than they are. Both terms are transparent intertextual references referring to the symptoms experienced by the patient. The third syndrome, however, is not a literature-inspired reference but a metaphor related to chess. *Knight's move thinking*, also known as *derailment*, is characterized by a disordered discourse, thus making reference to the way in which the knight moves in chess. Nevertheless, the culture tag is also understood in a more specific sense for disorders that have only been reported in certain countries or cultures (culture-bound syndromes), such as *koro*, *amok*, *piblokto*, etc. Another cause of variation is domain-based. For instance, *expressive aphasia* is also known as *Broca's aphasia* in clinical neuropsychology and as *agrammatic* aphasia in cognitive neuropsychology. Conceptual variation is also commonly found in the psychiatry domain, as in the example of echolalia, which may be regarded as a disorder-related symptom only if it occurs in adults.

These data categories and fields were drawn up following a top-down approach at the beginning of the research project. However, when it comes to compiling all these data for each concept and term, a corpus-based methodology must be devised. In the next section I describe three different approaches to explore the corpus.

3 Corpus-based analysis of dimensional variants

A specialized 10 million-word corpus was compiled for the Psychiatry domain in order to study different factors underlying term variation. It was divided according to user and genre types: expert, semi-specialized and encyclopaedic-didactic. The expert corpus contains specialized books and journal papers written by experts for experts, such as the *Diagnostic and Statistical Manual of Mental Disorders* (American Psychiatric Association, 2013). The semi-specialized corpus consists of web pages and brochures written by experts from Medline Plus and the National Institute of Mental Health, which combines basic and clinical research with information for patients, or their relatives, who suffer from any kind of mental disorder. Finally, the encyclopaedic-didactic corpus consists of a Wikipedia dump which was automatically collected through categories such as *Psychiatry*, *Syndromes*, *Disorders*, etc. I considered that Wikipedia should belong to this corpus because, being an encyclopaedic resource aimed at the overall comprehension of concepts, it usually contains metalinguistic information on synonyms and variants that could be useful in our research.

First of all, a semi-automatic procedure based on local grammars was designed in the NLP tool NooJ (Silberztein 2003) in order to extract term variants (León-Araúz and Reimerink 2014). Once the variant structures were extracted, I collected from the corpus all the concepts that showed more than one dimensional variant type and classified their corresponding forms according to the dimension conveyed. In Table 2-2, I show the dimensions I found with an illustrative example, which shows that term variation is often based on the same features that characterize the domain category of mental disorders.

Dimension	***Term variant***
+Discoverer	Korsakoff's psychosis
+Symptom	burning-mouth syndrome
+Cause	alcohol-induced amnestic disorder
+Body_part	teeth grinding
+Patient	boxer's dementia
+Result	bedwetting
+Intensity	mild cognitive impairment
+Time	short-term insomnia
+Location	prison psychosis

Table 2-2: Dimensional variant types found in the psychiatric corpus

Of course, there are variants that may show different dimensions at the same time, such as *chronic* [+Time] *traumatic* [+Cause] *brain* [+Body_part] *injury associated with boxing* [+Cause] or *alcohol-induced* [+Cause] *amnestic* [+Symptom] *disorder*. And there are also different variants for the same concept that highlight the same dimension, such as *Alice in Wonderland* [+Symptom] *syndrome* and *Lilliputian hallucination* [+Symptom], which refer to the same symptom of the disorder; or *nonsense* [+Symptom] *syndrome* and *syndrome of approximate answers* [+Symptom], which convey the same dimension but refer to two different symptoms.

Terminological resources should specify the conceptual dimension conveyed by each variant so that users could make a cognitively sound choice. However, from a cognitive point of view, the choice of one dimensional variant over the rest may also be related to the type of adjacent concepts activated in the discourse. Moreover, term choice also depends on communicative situations, namely, the expert-lay continuum. Therefore, term entries should also add use-related information. In what follows I propose a top-down three-phase methodology in order to analyse the correlation among different factors underlying term variation: (1) conceptual dimensions and text types (3.1), (2) term variants and text types (3.2), and (3) term variants' collocational context and text types (3.3).

3.1 Dimensions and text types

This analysis was carried out in order to find generalized patterns in the comparison of the three corpora with regards to the prevalence of dimensions. For this reason, as a further step, I annotated each dimensional variant type in the corpus (73 concept entries associated with 326 term variants) and performed new queries based on four of the most relevant dimensions found in the domain (Figure 2-3): +Discoverer, +Cause, +Symptom, +Body_part.

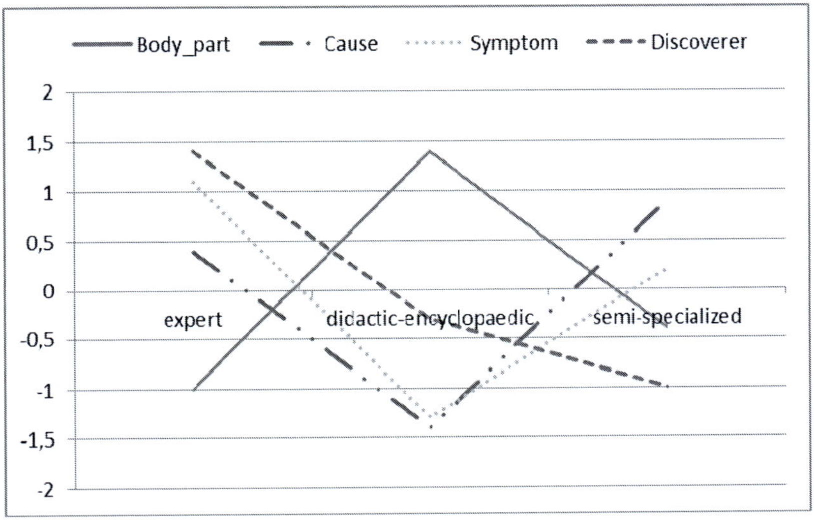

Fig. 2-3: Correlation of dimensional variants with the three corpora: +Discoverer; +Cause; +Symptom; and +Body_part

According to a patient-oriented approach, one might think at first that the +Symptom and +Body_part dimensions would be more semi-specialized than expert-related. However, surprisingly enough, it seems that the +Body_part dimension is only significant in the Wikipedia corpus, whereas the +Symptom dimension is most often found in the expert corpus as compared to the semi-specialized corpus. While in the expert corpus +Discoverer is the most prevalent dimension, +Symptom and +Cause are also significantly represented. As for the semi-specialized corpus, +Cause and +Symptom dimensions are most prototypical, inversely proportional as compared to the expert corpus.

Generally speaking, we can conclude that when there are competing variants, the translator should generally go for the eponym in expert settings, whereas in semi-specialized communication the cause-related term is the preferred option. Nevertheless, this is only a first approach to the study of cognitive and communicative correlation that should be further extended to a higher number of variants and other medical domains, since results can change dramatically when comparing domain-based differences. In this sense, Tsuji and Kageura (1998) observed in a medical corpus that person or virus names were more dominant than other variant types. In order to complement these findings, the different variants of the same concept were also individually studied. First, I studied their distribution in the corpora (see Section 3.2) and then I took a bottom-up manual approach to analyse their collocational context (see Section 3.3).

3.2 Term variants and text types

When querying the corpus, we observe that the variant *dementia pugilistica* is much more often used in the expert corpus as compared to *punchdrunk syndrome* or *boxer's dementia*. In this case, the Latin origin of the term points to the usual preference in expert settings. However, this preference is not always as straightforward. In such cases, users should have this information at hand. For instance, in Figure 2-4 three different variants for the same concept are represented according to usage-based preferences: *postnatal depression*, *postpartum depression*, and *baby blues*.

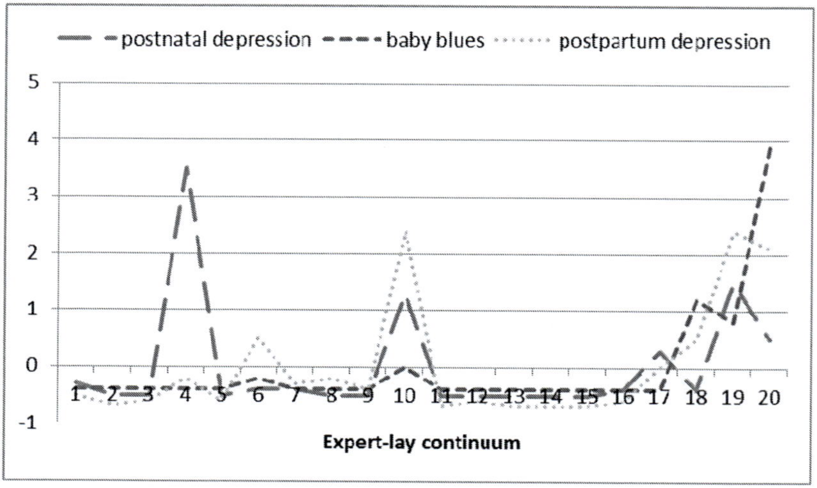

Fig. 2-4: Usage-based preferences for *baby blues*; *postpartum depression*; *postnatal depression*.

Strictly speaking, *baby blues* and *postpartum depression* are not fully synonyms. *Baby blues* is a milder version of *postpartum depression*, which lasts less time and has a much higher prevalence. However, the terms are often used synonymously, especially in semi-specialized texts, as their difference is a matter of degree rather than of kind. Since the aim of VariMed is to study all possible variants from a descriptive approach, they have been included in the same entry.

For this analysis, the three corpora were merged into a single file in order to observe these preferences as a continuum. In Figure 2-4, the first third of the graph represents the expert corpus, the second the Wikipedia corpus and the third the semi-specialized corpus. In NooJ, a single file corpus is automatically divided in twenty parts. This was done in order to observe more fine-grained peaks in which the three terms would occur or co-occur, since a corpus with three separate files would have drawn a less informative three-point graph. Not surprisingly, *baby blues* is the preferred term in semi-specialized communication, although the other two variants are also commonly found, as shown by the other peaks of the standard score graph. At first, *postnatal* and *postpartum depression* would seem interchangeable choices, but corpus analysis indicates that the use of one term or the other imposes a strong constraint on the communicative situation. *Postpartum depression* seems to be a more neutral term most often found in the Wikipedia didactic-encyclopaedic corpus and *postnatal depression* is the preferred term in expert texts.

3.3 Term variants and collocational context

This last phase was carried out in order to find out whether the activation of one term variant over the rest would also correlate with the type of concepts activated in their collocational context. This is in line with Bowker (1998), who states that the structure of the term (i.e. word order) used by an author is often influenced by the dimension that is considered the most significant to the discussion at hand. Her analysis focuses on the morphological term variants of *colour flatbed scanner* and *flatbed colour scanner*. She hypothesized (and proved true) that the author who is primarily concerned with the scanner's colour capability would refer to the concept as a *colour flatbed scanner*, while the author who is primarily interested in the scanner's design would refer to the same concept as a *flatbed colour scanner*. In this case, I collected and analysed 635 knowledge-rich contexts (KRCs) where all the term variants of the concept POSTPARTUM DEPRESSION occurred.[1] This concept was chosen because it was one of the few that showed representative results in the corpus in all of its forms. At this stage I also included its two acronyms (*PPD*, *PND*).

In Tables 2-3, 2-4, and 2-5 different KRCs have been included for illustrating the type of concepts co-occurring with *postnatal depression*, *postpartum depression* and *baby blues* in the expert, didactic-

[1] The name *knowledge-rich context* was introduced by Meyer (2001) for fragments retrieved from the corpus that are meaningful enough to show how the searched concept conceptually relates to others.

encyclopaedic and semi-specialized corpora respectively, as they are the most prototypical variants in each of the corpora. In the analysis, the co-occurring concepts (bold-faced in the tables) were assigned to broader conceptual categories (in small caps), such as TYPE (referring to hyperonyms like clinical depression), TREATMENT (both drugs and psychotherapy), PATIENT (women), DIAGNOSIS (assessment tools and scales, such as the Edinburgh Postnatal Scale or ICD diagnostic criteria), CAUSE (the baby, hormonal changes), TIME (after childbirth), SYMPTOM (crying, sleep disturbances), RESULT (negative behaviour), etc.

***postnatal depression* (expert corpus)**
DIAGNOSIS The **EPDS** has been extensively used to **screen** for *postnatal depression* in research and clinical practice in New Zealand.
DIAGNOSIS + PATIENT the accuracy of **assessment tools** for **depression** used in **women** with *postnatal depression* was fairly consistent with results reported for their use in general primary care settings.
DIAGNOSIS + TYPE **Depressive disorder** is used to refer to a condition meeting **DSM** or **ICD diagnostic criteria** for a **depressive disorder** (eg, major depression, dysthymia, *postnatal depression*).
DIAGNOSIS + SYMPTOM The GDT notes that the **EPDS** and **HADS** both **identify anxiety symptoms**, which are prominent in *postnatal depression.*
CAUSE + PATIENT there may be distinct **causative factors** for *postnatal depression* occurring in **women** with no history of a mood disorder (i.e., de novo), possibly associated with **postnatal neuroendocrine changes** A systematic review of literature on **risk factors** for *postnatal depression* found that potentially important factors were the **mother's level of social support, life events** and **psychiatric history**. **Women** with a **history of depressive disorders** may be at greater **risk** of developing *postnatal depression.*
TREATMENT **Nonpharmacological interventions** such as **enhanced social support** and/or a **psychological intervention** should be considered before prescribing **medication** for antenatal or *postnatal depression.*

Table 2-3: KRCs of *postnatal depression* in the expert corpus

***postpartum depression* (didactic encyclopaedic corpus)**
SYMPTOM + PATIENT **Unwanted thoughts** by **mothers** about **harming their newborn** infants are common in *postpartum depression* common **obsessions** about **harming babies** in **mothers** experiencing *postpartum depression* include **images of the baby lying dead in a casket or being eaten by sharks; stabbing the baby; throwing the baby down the stairs**;
SYMPTOM + PATIENT + TIME *Postpartum depression* occurs in **women after they have carried a child. Symptoms** include **sadness, fatigue, changes in sleeping and eating patterns, reduced libido, crying episodes, anxiety, and irritability**.
TYPE + PATIENT + TIME *Postpartum depression* is a type of **clinical depression** which can affect **women**, and less frequently **men**, typically **after childbirth**.
RESULT **Attachment**, **self-control** and other important **developmental attributes** are likely to be **disrupted in children of depressed mothers**. Furthermore, *postpartum depression* can predict **negative behavior in children** even years later.
PATIENT + TIME *Postpartum depression*, which affects 10–15% of **women**, typically sets in **within three months of childbirth**, and **lasts as long as three months**.

Table 2-4: KRCs of *postpartum depression* in the didactic-encyclopaedic corpus

***baby blues* (semi-specialized corpus)**
SYMPTOM If you have the *baby blues*, you may have **mood swings, feel sad, anxious or overwhelmed, have crying spells, lose your appetite, or have trouble sleeping**. Signs of the *baby blues* include **being teary, irritable or oversensitive** in your interactions with others, and having lots of **mood changes**.
TIME *Baby blues* may be experienced **after childbirth**.
SYMPTOM + TIME + CAUSE They commonly experience what is called the *baby blues*, **mood swings** that are the result of **high hormonal fluctuations** that occur during and immediately **after childbirth**.
SYMPTOM + TIME + CAUSE + PATIENT ...of **mood swings, tearfulness, anxiety and difficulty in sleeping** in the first week **after the birth** of a baby. Some 50-80% of **women** have such an experience. This episode, known as the *baby blues*, is thought to be linked with the **stresses associated with late pregnancy, labour and delivery**, along with the **rapid hormonal changes** that accompany the birth. Symptoms generally settle during the **first week after birth** **Women** with the *baby blues* may **feel tearful and overwhelmed**, due to **changes in hormone levels following childbirth**.

Table 2-5: KRCs of *baby blues* in the semi-specialized corpus

The different KRCs included in these tables show how the type of concept surrounding each variant changes across the three corpora. For instance, in the expert corpus *postnatal depression* is accompanied by concepts belonging to the categories of DIAGNOSIS and TREATMENT. In contrast, in the semi-specialized corpus, *baby blues* is most often surrounded by SYMPTOM-related concepts. However, there is also another factor driving this conceptual shift, which is that of term choice regardless of the corpus type. Therefore, as a further step, we compared the conceptual categories surrounding each variant within each of the corpora. Table 2-6 summarizes the results of analysing the 635 KRCs with regards to dimensions, degree of transparency, conceptual categories and text type. The degree of transparency was based on a 3-grade scale proposed by Gilreath (1993) to account for term descriptiveness, where 1 is transparent (highly descriptive), 2 is translucent (partly descriptive) and 3 is opaque (non-descriptive).

Variant	***Dimension***	***Transp.***	***Expert***	***Didactic-encyclopaedic***	***Semi-specialized***
postpartum depression	+Time	2	**Treatment** Cause **Patient** Time Result Diagnosis	**Symptom** Type Time Result **Patient**	Patient Time Cause **Symptom** Type Result **Treatment**
PPD	+Time	3		Type **Patient** Cause **Treatment** Time	Patient **Time** Type **Result** Symptom Cause
postnatal depression	+Time	2	Type **Cause** Treatment **Diagnosis**	**Type** **Time** Patient Cause Symptom	Result Type Symptom **Time** Patient
PND	+Time	3	Treatment **Diagnosis**		Patient **Symptom** Cause
baby blues	+Cause	1	**Symptom** Time		**Symptom** Cause **Time** Patient

Table 2-6: Correlation among variant type, dimension, transparency, KRCs and text type

The table includes the conceptual categories to which all co-occurring concepts belong, but there are certain categories that are more often activated than others in each case (bold-faced). The choice of *postpartum depression* seems to be significantly more related to the dimensions of TREATMENT, PATIENT and SYMPTOM in all text types. In contrast, *baby blues* appears clearly more related to the categories of SYMPTOM and TIME. On the other hand, *postnatal depression* seems to activate a totally different set of categories, which are CAUSE, TYPE, TIME and DIAGNOSIS. *PPD* shares with *postpartum depression* the categories of TREATMENT and PATIENT but adds two others, namely TIME and RESULT. *PND* is also related most often to a different category (SYMPTOM) as compared to its full form *postnatal depression*.

The difference between acronyms and their full forms might be related to the fact that acronyms are usually activated in the text after full forms. Thus, the logical order in which the disorder is described might condition the category types accompanying acronyms. *Postpartum depression* and *postnatal depression* are the only term variants that are representative enough in all the three corpora. They are also the terms that co-occur with the highest number of categories (8). The acronym *PPD* is hardly ever found in the expert corpus (maybe because, in psychiatry, it can also mean *paranoid personality disorder*), whereas the acronym *PND* is never found in the didactic-encyclopaedic corpus.

If we go into more detail, we can observe that there are also certain preference patterns related to text type. For instance, the conceptual categories activated in the context of *postpartum depression* change across the expert-lay continuum. Even though there are certain categories present in all three corpora (e.g. RESULT and TIME), only one significant category (bold-faced) overlaps at a time: in the expert corpus, significant categories are TREATMENT and PATIENT; the second category, PATIENT, is also significantly found in the didactic-encyclopaedic corpus together with the SYMPTOM category; which is also shared by the semi-specialized corpus together with the TREATMENT category (as in the expert corpus). In *postnatal depression*, however, only the TIME category is common to the didactic-encyclopaedic and semi-specialized corpora. The rest of the significant categories vary across text types. Finally, in the case of *baby blues*, the category that is most often encountered is SYMPTOM, regardless of the text type where it occurs.

If we focus in one text type only, term choice appears not only to depend on text types and register-based preferences, but also on conceptually-dependent collocates. For instance, within the expert corpus the choice of *postpartum depression* or *postnatal depression* activates a different set of significant categories (TREATMENT and PATIENT vs. DIAGNOSIS and CAUSE).

4 Conclusion

In this paper I have shown how term variants in the psychiatric domain are cognitive and communicatively motivated. From a cognitive perspective, variants reflect the prototypical dimensions in which psychiatric disorders may be classified. Furthermore, the dimensions activated in their collocational context show that the use of one variant or the other implies a different cognitive and pragmatic positioning. From a communicative perspective, terms and dimensions can also be associated with user-based parameters. However, further studies need to be done with regards to the correlation between the cognitive and communicative factors underlying term variation, especially from a cross-linguistic perspective, since not all cultures conceptualize specialized domains in the same way, nor do they address their audience in the same manner. Sometimes, expert variants do not match the same conceptual dimensions activated in their formal counterpart in other languages. Therefore, translators need access to meaningful terminological knowledge bases so as to strike a balance between conceptual information and register-based preferences.

Acknowledgements

This study was carried out within the framework of the R&D project VARIMED (FFI2011-23120) funded by the Spanish Ministry of Education, Culture and Sports.

References

American Psychiatric Association (2013), *Diagnostic and statistical manual of mental disorders*, 5th ed., Arlington (VA): American Psychiatric Publishing.

Bowker, Lynne (1997), 'Multidimensional Classification of Concepts and Terms', in Wright, Sue Ellen & Budin Gerhard (eds.) *Handbook of Terminology Management Volume 1: Basic Aspects of Terminology Management*, Amsterdam: John Benjamins, 133-143.

—. (1998), 'Variant terminology: frivolity or necessity?', in Fontenelle, T., Hiligsmann P., Michiels A., Moulin A. & Theissen S. (eds.), *Proceedings of EURALEX' 98*, Liège: University of Liège, 487-495.

Bowker, Lynne & Hawkins Shane (2006), 'Variation in the organization of medical terms: Exploring some motivations for term choice', *Terminology* 12 (1):79-110.

Candel Mora, Miguel Ángel & Carrió Pastor, Marisa (2012), 'Corpus analysis: A pragmatic perspective on term variation', *Revista Española de Lingüística Aplicada* 1:33-50.

Fernández-Silva, Sabela (2010), *Variación Terminológica y Cognición. Factores Cognitivos en la Denominación del Concepto Especializado*, PhD Thesis, Barcelona: Universitat Pompeu Fabra.

Fernández-Silva, Sabela; Freixa, Judit & Cabré, María Teresa (2011), 'A Proposed Method for Analysing the Dynamics of Cognition through Term Variation', *Terminology* 17 (1):49-73.

Fernández-Silva, Sabela; Freixa, Judit & Cabré, María Teresa (2014), 'A proposed method for analysing the dynamics of naming from a intralingual and interlingual perspective', in Temmerman, R. & Van Campenhoudt, M. (eds.), *The dynamics of culture-bound terminology in monolingual and multilingual communication*, Amsterdam: John Benjamins.

Freixa, Judit (2006), 'Causes of Denominative Variation in Terminology: A Typology Proposal', *Terminology* 12 (1):51-77.

—. (2002), *La Variació terminològica: Anàlisi de la variació denomitiva en textos de different grau d'especialització de l'àrea de medi ambient*, PhD Thesis, Barcelona: University of Barcelona.

Gilreath, Charles (1993), 'Onometrics: the formal evaluation of terms', in Strehlow, R. A. & Wright, S. E. (eds.), *Standardizing Terminology for Better Communication: Practice, Applied Theory, and Results*, Philadelphia (PA): ASTM, 75-95.

Gregory, Michael & Carroll, Suzanne (1978), *Language and situation: Language varieties and their social contexts*, London: Routledge and Kegan Paul.

Kageura, Kyo (1997), 'Multifaceted/Multidimensional Concept Systems', in Wright, S. E. & Budin G. (eds.), *Handbook of Terminology Management: Basic Aspects of Terminology Management*, Amsterdam: John Benjamins, 119-132.

León-Araúz, Pilar & Reimerink, Arianne (2014), 'From term dynamics to concept dynamics: term variation and multidimensionality in the psychiatric domain', in Abel, A., Vettori C., and Ralli, N. (eds.), *Proceedings of EURALEX'14*, Bolzano: EURAC, 657-668.

León-Araúz, Pilar; Reimerink, Arianne & Aragón, Alejandro G. (2013), 'Dynamism and context in specialized knowledge', *Terminology* 19 (1): 31-61.

Merkel, Magnus (1996), 'Consistency and Variation in Technical Translations a Study of Translators' Attitudes', in Proceedings of *Unity in Diversity, International Translation Studies Conference*. Dublin City University, 9-11 May 1996.
http://www.ida.liu.se/~magme/publications/dublin.pdf
(accessed 2 Feb. 2015).

Meyer, Ingrid (2001), 'Extracting Knowledge-Rich Contexts for Terminography: A conceptual and methodological framework', in Bourigault, Didier; Jacquemin, Christian & L'Homme, Marie-Claude (eds.), *Recent Advances in Computational Terminology*, Amsterdam: John Benjamins, 279-302.

Picht, Heribert & Draskau, Jennifer (1985), *Terminology: An Introduction*, Guildford: University of Surrey.

Rogers, Margaret (1997), 'Synonymy and Equivalence in Special-Language Texts: A Case Study in German and English Texts on Genetic Engineering', in Trosborg A. (ed.), *Text Typology and Translation*, Amsterdam: John Benjamins, 217-246.

Rogers, Margaret (2004), 'Multidimensionality in Concepts Systems: A Bilingual Textual Perspective', *Terminology* 10 (2): 215-240.

Silberztein,Max (2003), 'NooJ Manual', http://www.nooj4nlp.net/NooJManual.pdf (viewed 6 Feb. 2015).

Tercedor Sánchez, María Isabel; López Rodríguez, Clara Inés; Prieto Velasco, Juan Antonio (2014), 'También los pacientes hacen terminología: retos del proyecto VariMed', *Panace@: Revista de Medicina, Lenguaje y Traducción*, 15 (39): 95-102.

Tsuji, Keita & Kageura, Kyo (1998), 'An analysis of medical synonyms: The word-structure of preferred terms', *Terminology* 5(2):229-249.

Wright, Sue Ellen (1997), 'Representation of Concept Systems', in Wright, Sue Ellen & Budin Gerhard (eds.), *Handbook of Terminology Management: Basic Aspects of Terminology Management*, Amsterdam: John Benjamins, 89-97.

CHAPTER THREE

NAMING DEVICES IN MIDDLE-EAR SURGERY: A MORPHOLOGICAL ANALYSIS

PIUS TEN HACKEN

The middle ear is the area of the ear between the eardrum and the inner ear. It contains three tiny bones called *ossicles*, which play a central role in the transfer of sound between the eardrum and the cochlea. It is linked to the nose by the Eustachian tube. Middle-ear surgery is a highly specialized area of medicine. Here I will present a morphological analysis of the terminology found in a specialized handbook, Gersdorff & Gérard (2011), which describes the anatomy, surgical instruments and surgical operations. Section 1 presents the handbook and the field, as well as the terminology collection process. Section 2 gives an overview of the morphological structure of the terms in the collection. Section 3 analyses the correlation between morphological structure and transparency of the terms. Section 4 summarizes the main outcomes of the analysis and suggests an interpretation.

1 The Handbook of Middle-Ear Surgery

The collection of terms to be analysed here is determined by a single handbook of the domain, Gersdorff & Gérard (2011). According to its title, this book is an atlas. It is a relatively slim volume (136 pages for the main text) with large pages (310 x 230 mm, larger than DIN A4) and many images (254). The images are drawings, sometimes including arrows to indicate movement. Large portions of the book consist only of images and captions, and continuous texts of more than 200 words are very rare. The authors are two medical specialists affiliated with the Clinique Universitaire St. Luc (Brussels) and the Université Catholique de Louvain (Louvain-la-Neuve), both French-speaking institutions in Belgium. There is no indication that the text has been translated.

As stated in the foreword, "[t]his book is written for the otorhinolaryngologist" (2011: v). The first three chapters can be considered introductory. Chapter 1 gives an overview of the anatomy of the middle-ear (2011: 1-5). Here we find images of the type familiar from visual dictionaries such as Corbeil & Archambault (1997), where terms are linked to a named portion of the image by a line. Chapter 2 describes the anesthesia and the organization of the operation room (2011: 7-10). Chapter 3 presents the surgical tools (2011: 11-16). The core of this chapter is a set of 29 images of instruments with their names in the captions. These chapters are very brief, especially if we consider that the first page of each is only a title page. Most of the information is conveyed by means of images.

The next three chapters address the actions performed in the medical operations. They constitute the core of the book (2011: 17-133). In these chapters, the pages have a layout with two vertically arranged print areas. The larger one, 135 mm wide, is closer to the spine and normally contains two figures, one above the other. Occasionally we find brief texts, mostly 3-7 lines, in this area as well. The narrower area, 55 mm wide, is grey underlaid and contains text explaining the figures. It also contains headings to facilitate quick navigation. There are three levels of headings, the lowest is used as a title for each figure. There are also practical tips for the surgeon interrupting the grey columns. They are in blue on a light-blue background. This layout is also visible in other chapters, but not applied as consistently as here.

Chapter 7 describes postoperative care (2011: 135-136). It has 13 lines of text and no images. After the main text, there is an index (2011: 137-140). Before the main text, there are two forewords recommending the work and two prefaces by the two authors. The forewords and prefaces were not considered in the terminology collection.

Term extraction was done manually. The source was not available in electronic form, but even if it had been, there are various reasons why manual term extraction is to be preferred in a case like this. With 747 terms (types), the density is very high. Excluding title pages and blank pages, the book has 126 pages, so that we found almost 6.0 new terms per page on average. Given the small amount of text per page, this is a remarkable density. We did not count the tokens, but in an atlas of this kind, the type/token ratio is high. As soon as one area with its terms has been introduced, attention is directed to the next area, so that for many terms there is little opportunity to repeat them.

Most if not all terms in the sample belong to what in ten Hacken (2015a) is called *specialized vocabulary*. The alternative, *terms in the narrow sense*, requires a precise definition with necessary and sufficient conditions, which is only necessary in case the exact classification of borderline cases is significant. In medicine, this may occur when insurance cover has to be determined or when scientific claims are made. However, Gersdorff & Gérard's (2011) atlas is rather a practical aid for surgeons, so that these perspectives are not prominent.

In selecting terms, we did not attempt to make any domain classification. In general, medical terminology is marked by a large degree of specialization. At the same time, a particular text will typically contain terminology from several medical domains and degrees of specialization. Thus, the surgical tools in chapter 3 are not necessarily limited to middle-ear surgery. The collection of terms contains all medical terms found in Gersdorff & Gérard's (2011) atlas.

2 Morphological Structure

A good measure to express the morphological complexity of the terms is the number of stems involved. In the terms in our collection, this number ranges from 1 to 5. Fig. 3-1 gives a breakdown of the total set into these five classes.

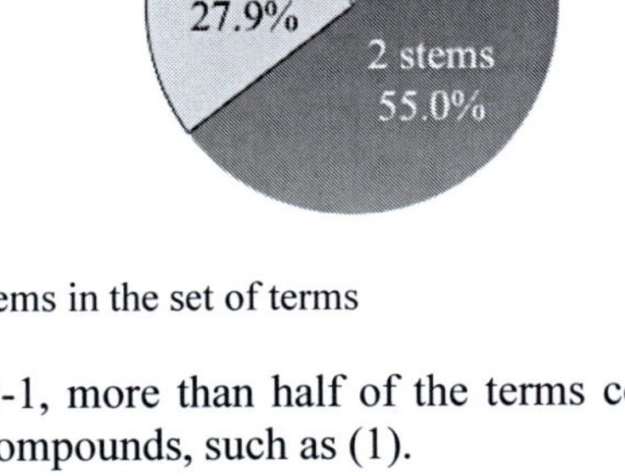

Fig.3-1: Number of stems in the set of terms

As shown in Fig. 3-1, more than half of the terms consist of two stems. Many of these are compounds, such as (1).

(1) a. stapes arch
    b. incus erosion

By concentrating on the number of stems, I consciously ignore the complexity of the stem. Thus, (1b) is counted as having two stems, although *erosion* consists of two morphemes. This raises the question of where to draw the line between affixes and stems. This question is particularly acute for neoclassical formations. There are a number of terms ending in *-plasty*, such as (2).

(2) a. ossiculoplasty
b. tympanoplasty

There is no word **plasty* in English, but the element clearly contains a stem. In line with the analysis I propose in ten Hacken (2012), one can assume that there is a bound stem *plast(o)*, which has to combine with an affix in order to get a syntactic category so that it can be used in a sentence. In (2), it first combines with the bound stems *ossiculo* and *tympano* to form a compound, which subsequently becomes a noun when affixed with *-y*.

Whereas it is obvious that *-y* in (2) is an affix, as well as *-ion* in (1b), there are also more problematic cases. In the case of *-y* and *-ion*, the suffix only determines the syntactic category. Prefixes often have a more prominent meaning, as in (3).

(3) a. perilymphatic
b. epitympanic

The prefixes *peri-* in (3a) and *epi-* in (3b) correspond to Ancient Greek prepositions. As opposed to the stem *tympan(o)* in (2b) and (3b), which can be the first or the second morpheme, prefixes such as *epi-* can only appear when followed by a stem. Therefore, the cases in (3) were counted as having one stem.

It is well known that for languages like English, orthographic words do not give reliable evidence for the nature of the morphological construction. We even find minimal pairs such as in (4).

(4) a. eardrum [Gersdorff & Gérard (2011: 27)]
b. ear drum [Gersdorff & Gérard (2011: 30)]

Rather than assuming that (4a) or (4b) is an error, the occurrence of both in different contexts suggests that this aspect of the spelling is not fixed in the case of this term. The fact that such cases occur is a further reason why a division according to stems is more fruitful than one according to orthographic words.

By counting stems we cannot determine the construction. The contrast illustrated in (5) is a case in point.

(5) a. fixed speculum
b. nasal speculum

In both (5a) and (5b), we have an adjective modifying a noun. However, whereas *fixed* in (5a) is a qualitative adjective, *nasal* is a relational adjective (RA). In (5a), *fixed* designates a property of *speculum*, but in (5b), *nasal* expresses a relationship to the noun *nose*. As argued by, for instance, Levi (1978), ten Hacken (1994, 2013), there are good reasons to classify RA+N constructions such as (5b) as compounds. The RA+N combination should be analysed as a morphological construction intended for word formation, whereas A+N constructions of the type illustrated in (5a) are syntactically formed.

A detailed breakdown of the terms with two stems is given in Fig. 3-2.

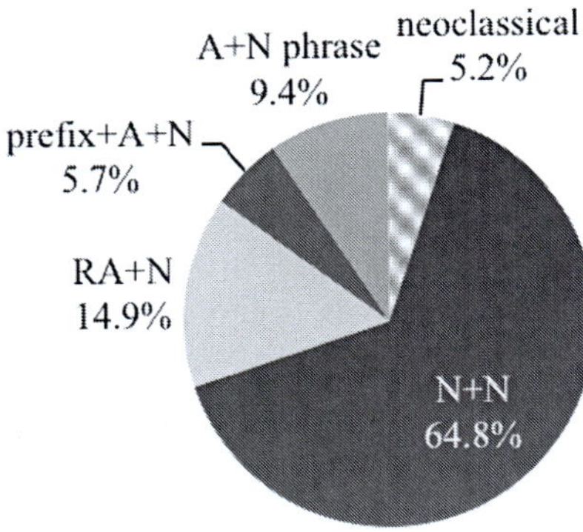

Fig. 3-2: Types of terms with two stems

As shown in Fig. 3-2, almost two thirds of the terms with two stems are N+N compounds. If we accept cases such as (5b) with a relational adjective as compounds as well, the proportion of compounds rises to almost 80%. The neoclassical category includes cases such as (2). They are often called neoclassical compounds and semantically they behave in much the same way as N+N compounds. The category labeled as 'prefix+A+N' includes cases such as (6).

(6) a. epidermal migration
b. retroauricular incision
c. anti-Trendelenburg position

In (6a-b) we find a neoclassical adjective with a prefix. The stem in (6a) is *derma(to)* ('skin') and the adjective means 'across the skin'. In (6b), the stem is *auricul(o)* ('ear') and the adjective means 'behind the ear'. Whereas (6a) is composed of Ancient Greek elements, (6b) is from Latin elements. In both cases, a prefix is attached to what in the classical language is a nominal stem. In (6c), we find the same basic structure but with an eponym as the stem. As I argue in ten Hacken (2003), it is not really possible to determine the syntactic category of the non-head of a compound, because this element is not syntactically active. If we assume that (6c) is a compound, it is reasonable to extend such an analysis to (6a-b). It is only A+N phrases, illustrated by (5a), which cannot be considered compounds. As shown in Fig.3-2, they make up less than 10%.

For obvious reasons, the set of terms with only one stem, which makes up almost 10% of the total set, does not contain compounds. Some typical examples from this set are given in (7).

(7) a. antrum
b. curette
c. microsuction
d. epithelialization

Some, but certainly not all terms with one stem show derivation. In (7a), we see a case of an underived loanword. *Antrum* means 'cave' in Latin and is used to designate particular types of cavities in medical English. In (7b), it may be thought that we have an instance of the suffix *-ette*. Marchand (1969: 289-91) treats *-ette* as a suffix and gives the example of *kitchenette* to demonstrate that it has been used as a word formation device in English. Given that *curette* does not mean 'a small cure', but refers to a surgical instrument, we do not have a derivational base for such an analysis in English. Bauer et al. . (2013: 395) state about *-ette* that "[i]t is no longer productive on bound bases." One of their examples is *camionette*. In fact, it is more plausible that *camionette* and *curette* were borrowed from French independently of the French base, which was not borrowed.

In (7c-d) we do have derivation. In (7c) the prefix *micro-* is used. Although this is an adjectival stem in Ancient Greek, it has developed into a prefix in English (cf. Bauer et al. 2013: 397). (7d) is a neoclassical formation. The Ancient Greek stem θηλή ('nipple') is combined with the prefix *epi-* to form *epithelium*, a type of thin skin. Then suffixation with *-al* gives the adjective corresponding to this noun and suffixation with *-ize* gives *epithelialize*, the verb referring to 'the formation of epithelium'. The term is normally cited in its nominalized form with *-ation*, which constitutes a transposition (cf. ten Hacken, 2015b).

When we turn to longer terms, we do not find any new process types. Some examples of terms with three stems are given in (8).

(8) a. eustachian tube closure
b. small-diameter suction
c. tympanomeatal flap

All of the examples in (8) can easily be recognized as compounds. The difference in structure concerns only the non-head. In (8a), the non-head is a compound consisting of a relational adjective and a noun. In (8b), *small diameter* is a phrasal combination. It is not itself a term, but it is used to qualify the head *suction*. In (8c) the non-head is a neoclassical compound that appears as a relational adjective. Some examples of longer terms are given in (9).

(9) a. short process axis continuity
b. anterior meatal skin flap
c. xenogenous graft tympanoplasty

In each of the examples in (9), there is at least one adjectival component, but this does not automatically lead to a phrasal structure. In (9a), *short process* is a phrase, but it is embedded in the non-head of a compound. We will return to the structure of (9b) in section 3 below. In (9c), *xenogenous* is the adjectival form of a neoclassical compound. It combines with *graft* as the phrasal non-head of a compound.

In general, we can say that the large majority of terms in our sample should be classified as compounds. Some 10% contain only one stem and can therefore not be compounds. Among terms with two stems, we find some A+N phrases, but they are just over 5% of the total number of terms. Among longer terms, we find this A+N phrasal pattern as well, e.g. (9b), but it is rare. Among compounds, the N+N structure predominates, but RA+N is also quite frequent. With longer compounds, there tend to be more adjectival components, with most of them being relational adjectives, but also adjectives embedded in a phrasal non-head.

3 Transparency and Motivation

The question of the transparency of a complex word is tightly linked to what Saussure (1916: 100) called *l'arbitraire du signe*. When we consider a word as a Saussurean sign with a form (*signifiant*) and a meaning (*signifié*), the form is not determined by the meaning. The fact that the animal called *dog* in English is *hond* in Dutch, *cane* in Italian, and *pies* in

Polish illustrates this point. The arbitrariness does not mean that any speaker can make up a word for *dog*. In the English speech community, the word *dog* has long been established, so children learning English as their native language will get to know this word as the right one. This idea of a word being established in a speech community is one type of motivation. The Italian word *cane* can be motivated further by its etymological relationship to Latin *canis*. Also the Dutch word *hond* can be etymologically related to *canis*. There is a sound law correlating Latin /k/ and Germanic /h/, cf. Latin *cor*, Dutch *hart* ('heart'). Etymological relations provide another type of motivation. It can thus be argued that signs are in general not unmotivated. However, motivation is not the opposite of what Saussure intended with his *arbitraire du signe*.

As Saussure (1916: 180-82) realized, morphological relations reduce the degree of arbitrariness of a sign. He gives the example of complex numbers. English *nineteen* seems entirely transparent, because it designates the sum of nine and ten. However, French has *dix-neuf* (lit. 'ten-nine'), Latin *undeviginti* (lit. 'one from twenty') and Welsh *pedwar ar bymtheg* (lit. 'four and fifteen'). In *nineteen*, we can identify two types of arbitrariness. On one hand, *nine* and *ten* are arbitrary (though historically and socially motivated). This is a limitation of transparency. On the other hand, as the French, Latin and Welsh examples show, the way 19 is calculated is not determined by the outcome. This is a limitation of motivation. Whereas motivation represents an onomasiological perspective, as it relates to the speaker choosing a name, transparency is semasiologically oriented, related to the hearer interpreting the name.

In Jackendoff's (1975) proposal for the organization of the lexicon, redundancy rules are used to encode morphological relations. The idea is that *nineteen* has a lexical entry of its own, but that the relation to *nine* and *ten* reduces the impact on storage. What is stated in the entry for *nine* does not count in calculating the cost for storing *nineteen*. The cost of the entry for *nineteen* is then only the order of the two items, the references to the entries for *nine* and *ten* and the idiosyncratic vowel change of *ten* to *teen*. A further reduction can be achieved by the observation that the order of the items and the lengthening of the vowel in *ten* apply in the same way to numbers form thirteen to eighteen. The fact that the special rules for these numbers have a very limited scope means that the reduction they entail is more restricted than the references to *nine* and *ten*. In Jackendoff's model, this can be expressed by assuming that the reference to a rule costs more when the rule is more limited in scope.

What is encoded in redundancy rules is only transparency, not motivation. A redundancy rule states information that can be derived from a more general observation, i.e. information that applies to a larger class of lexical items. This information contributes to the transparency of a form. A redundancy rule does not state why a particular form is used. That would be the motivation for this form.

We can now apply these notions to the set of terms in middle-ear surgery. As a starting point, let us consider the examples in (7) again, repeated here as (10).

(10) a. antrum
b. curette
c. microsuction
d. epithelialization

As noted in section 2, (10a) is borrowed from Latin and (10b) from French. In both cases, the medical sense is an extension of a more basic sense, 'cave' for (10a) and 'scraper' for (10b). There is a difference, however, in the sense that *curette* was used in French in the same medical sense as in English before it was borrowed, whereas the sense extension of *antrum* to the medical sense was not carried out by native speakers of Latin. Of course, Latin was used in medicine for a long time when it no longer had any native speakers, so it is difficult to establish how exactly this sense of *antrum* in Latin relates to the English term.

The derivational analysis of (10c-d) was given in section 2. In order to evaluate the transparency of (10c), we need to analyse its meaning. Gersdorff & Gérard (2011: 12) use *microsuction* in the sentences in (11).

(11) a. Microsuction is used for the middle ear cavity and precise mastoid surgery.
b. Single-use microsuctions with a diameter less than 0.7 mm are used around fragile and precarious structures [...].

In (11a), *microsuction* is used to refer to a type of suction, i.e. the removal of fluid material by means of a vacuum. In this sense, *microsuction* is not countable. In (11b), which in the text immediately follows (11a), it appears in the plural. Here, it refers to an instrument, of which Gersdorff & Gérard (2011: 14) also give a picture.

In a lexicon of the type proposed by Jackendoff (1975), the two senses of *microsuction* are represented in separate entries. The entry for the process, used in (11a), can refer to *suction* and the prefix *micro-*. The remaining part of the meaning is very small. The entry for the medical instrument, used in (11b), can refer to the entry for the process. This covers the entire form, but significant further information has to be specified. Although the reference to the entry used in (11a) gives an indication of what the instrument does, there is no information about what the instrument looks like, how it works, etc. Moreover, the step from process to instrument is not very common, at least compared to the way how *micro-* affects the meaning of *suction* in the process reading of *microsuction*. Therefore, the cost of the entry for (10c) in the sense used in (11a) is quite low, but the cost for the sense used in (11b) is much higher.

In (10d), *epithelium* is a base that in the English lexicon is non-transparent. Compared to (10a-b), also its form is absent from the classical languages its components stem from. It is a neoclassical formation. As opposed to formations such as *morphology*, where both elements are readily recognizable because of their recurrence in other formations such as *anthropomorphic* and *anthropology*, the stem in *epithelium* does not occur elsewhere. Therefore its analysis is only etymologically relevant. The suffixation rules adding *-al*, *-ize* and *-ation* are very prominent in English. The entire form can be understood by any speaker of English who knows *epithelium*. This can be encoded by means of redundancy rules for the three suffixation processes. Therefore, the cost of the entry for (10d) is quite low, but the cost for the entry for *epithelium*, which it refers to, is much higher.

Let us now turn to compounding. As noted in section 2, compounding accounts for the large majority of terms considered here. There are a number of properties that generally make compounds less transparent than syntactic constructions. The contrast in (12) illustrates one of them.

(12) a. fascia graft
b. harvest graft

Both compounds in (12) have the head *graft*. A graft is a piece of tissue that is used for transplantation. In N+N compounds such as (12), it is not expressed how the non-head specifies the head. The relation has to be inferred on the basis of the meaning of the head, the meaning of the non-head and the context of use. This can lead to contrasts such as the one in (12). The contexts in (13) are taken from Gersdorff & Gérard (2011).

(13) a. Cleaning the fascia graft as much as possible before harvesting further facilitates fascia trimming. (2011: 19)
b. […], the harvest graft is taken from the posterior edge of the retroauricular incision, […] (2011: 26)

Whereas *fascia graft* indicates a piece of fascia (fibrous tissue) to be grafted, *harvest graft* indicates a piece of tissue that has been harvested so that it can be used for grafting. In (12a), the non-head indicates the nature of the tissue, whereas in (12b) it is the role of the tissue in the grafting procedure that is indicated. The only way to determine the different relationships between the head and the non-head is to know enough about the domain to infer that these are the intended relationships.

It is worth considering to what extent the relationship in a compound is determined by properties of the expression. In (14), a number of different types of compound and a phrasal expression are listed.

(14) a. retraction pocket
b. facial nerve
c. incus mobilization
d. fixed speculum

In (14a), we have an N+N compound similar to (12). The two nouns do not indicate what the relation between them is. In this case, *pocket* is used metaphorically to indicate an enclosed space and *retraction* expresses how this space is used. A retraction pocket is a place where epithelium concentrates, which may lead to a cholesteatoma.

In (14b), *facial* is a relational adjective. The main argument for considering RA+N combinations as compounds is that the way the relation between the two components is determined is the same as for N+N compounds. Of course the relation has to be determined for the underlying noun, *face* in (14b). In this case, the non-head indicates the place where the nerve is located. Again, this relation can only be inferred on the basis of domain knowledge. It is not overtly expressed.

The situation is slightly different in cases such as (14c). The reason is that the head incorporates a verb, *mobilize*. In the case of deverbal nouns in *-ation*, this results in a strong preference for the interpretation of the non-head as the object of the underlying verb (at least if the verb is transitive). The same applies to a number of other noun-forming suffixes, e.g. *-er* and *-ing*. Therefore, (14c) is more transparent than (14a-b) and (12). It is this property that made Roeper & Siegel (1978) propose a separate mechanism for such deverbal compounds, a proposal which triggered a range of alternative competing theories for this construction. It should be noted that the interpretation of the non-head as an object is only a preference. This is illustrated in (15).

(15) a. cartilage incision
b. Rosen incision

Whereas in (15a), *cartilage* serves as the object of *incise*, in the same way as *incus* in (14c), the role of *Rosen* in (15b) is different. We will come back to this example below.

The basic indeterminacy of the relation in compounds contrasts with the situation we find in phrasal expressions such as (14d). In contrast to the relational adjective in (14b), *fixed* does not specify a relation to a noun, but designates a property that is assigned to the referent identified by the head noun *speculum*.

In sum, we can say that the relationship between the components of a compound is not made explicit. This reduces their transparency. When the head of the compound is deverbal, transparency is less affected, because the verb can be expected to determine this relation. The difference in transparency is particularly obvious in the contrast between RA+N compounds and regular A+N phrases.

A second property that reduces the transparency of compounds is their lack of specification of the internal structure. An example is (16).

(16) a. incus mobility testing
 b. [incus [mobility testing]]
 c. [[incus mobility] testing]

The compound in (16a) has three basic components. Therefore, both structures in (16b-c) are possible. There is a relatively clear contrast in meaning associated with the contrast between these structures. In (16b), *mobility testing* is the name of the process involved, whereas in (16c) *incus mobility* describes what is tested. In this case, (16c) is the correct structure.

Ambiguities of the type illustrated in (16) only arise for compounds with three or more basic components. Given that compounding is a binary process, but at each stage the direction of combination can follow the pattern in (16b) or (16c), the number of potential structures rises steeply with each additional component. It does not matter whether a non-head component is a relational adjective or a noun. Even with certain other adjectives than relational ones, the structural ambiguity arises. This is illustrated in (17) for the term with four basic components given as (9b) above.

(17) a. anterior meatal skin flap
 b. [anterior [meatal [skin flap]]]
 c. [anterior [[meatal skin] flap]]
 d. [[anterior meatal] [skin flap]]
 e. [[anterior [meatal skin]] flap]
 f. [[[anterior meatal] skin] flap]

In terms of syntactic category, (17a) has two adjectives followed by two nouns. *Meatal* is a relational adjective corresponding to *meatus* ('passage'). In our domain it refers to the canal between the outer ear and the middle ear. *Anterior* is an inherent comparative. None of the five theoretically possible binary structures in (17b-f) can be excluded without resorting to world knowledge. Only the fact that the human body does not have anterior and posterior meatus is the basis for excluding (17d) and (17f), not any kind of prohibition for adjectives to modify a relational adjective. Their exclusion follows the same pattern of reasoning as the exclusion of (17e), where *anterior* is applied to *meatal skin*. A further illustration of this principle takes (18) as a basis.

(18) titanium total ossicular replacement prosthesis

With five components, (18) has fourteen possible binary structures. Like *anterior* in (17), *total* in (18) is a non-relational adjective. As shown by (18), such adjectives do not have to appear as first elements and can in fact be preceded by a noun. In addition, *ossicular* is a relational adjective. The fact that such highly ambiguous compounds can be used successfully in communication can be explained because much of the ambiguity is not noticed in practice. In reading (18), someone familiar with the field will first of all group together *ossicular replacement*, because it is a familiar concept. This reduces the number of structures to five, corresponding to the ambiguity in (17). In a next step, *total* is combined with *ossicular replacement*. This leaves only two possible structures, corresponding to the ambiguity in (16).

In sum, the structure of compounds with more than two basic components is ambiguous, because there are no formal indicators for it. The degree of ambiguity rapidly increases for longer compounds. Resolution of the ambiguity depends on world knowledge and proceeds through gradual reduction of the number of possibilities.

A final source of reduced transparency in compounds is the appearance of opaque components. In general, in order to understand a compound we need to know the meaning of its parts. To someone who does not know the meaning of *graft*, the compounds in (12) are not transparent. What I mean here, however, is that in some compounds there are components for which it does not help knowing what they refer to. One type of components to which this applies is proper names as in (19).

(19) a. Trendelenburg position
b. Rosen incision

Knowledge about the meaning of *Trendelenburg* does not contribute to understanding the meaning of (19a). Friedrich Trendelenburg (1844-1924) was a German surgeon, born in Berlin, who studied in Glasgow and Edinburgh and worked at the universities of Rostock, Bonn, and Leipzig. He was one of the founding fathers of the Deutsche Gesellschaft für Chirurgie ('German Society of Surgery'). However, any amount of biographic information about this person does not contribute to understanding the compound in (19a).

Compounds such as (19) are not compositional. In a model of the lexicon such as Jackendoff's (1975), a reference to the proper name is not cost-effective. For (19b), where I have not been able to identify the person referred to by *Rosen*, we are not at a disadvantage compared to (19a). In the case of (19), we need global information, i.e. a description of the particular position and the type of incision, rather than identification of the person referred to by the non-head.

Another type of opaque element is illustrated in (20).

(20) type 2 ossiculoplasty

The contribution of *type 2* in (20) to the meaning of the entire compound is of the same kind as the contribution of the proper names in (19). It can be assumed that, at some point, someone proposed a typology of ossiculoplasty with at least two types. In the original publication, the types were explained so that the name in (20) referred to an explicit classification. Perhaps this was Sadé (1988). Meanwhile, the individual types have been generally accepted and at least (20) has been established as a concept, as can be seen by its use in the title of medical articles, e.g. Felek et al. (2010). Gersdorff & Gérard (2011: 88) also use the term in (20) without any reference to a publication or to other types.

In sum, opaque elements directly affect the transparency of the compounds they appear in. The most common type is the proper name, used especially when a concept is named after its originator. Another type consists of arbitrary distinctions, numerical or otherwise, which become established as standard terms. In the original context of naming, these elements were not unmotivated, but the motivation is no longer accessible outside this context, so that it does not contribute to transparency.

A phenomenon that needs to be mentioned here is the interaction between the different sources of opacity. This is illustrated by (21).

(21) Henle spine protrusion

First, *Henle* is a proper name. It refers to Friedrich Gustav Jakob Henle (1809-1885), a German physician, pathologist and anatomist, who wrote an influential *Handbuch der systematischen Anatomie des Menschen* ('Handbook of Systematic Human Anatomy'). As in (19), this information does not contribute to the decoding of (21). However, (21) is also ambiguous in the same sense as (16). Whereas in (16) we only need to know which of the structures makes most sense, in (21) we have to find out whether a spine or a protrusion were named after Henle. In this case, the correct structure is the one parallel to (16c), with *Henle spine* as a constituent.

4 Morphology, Transparency and World Knowledge

In this chapter, I offered an analysis of the terminology in Gersdorff & Gérard's (2011) *Atlas of Middle Ear Surgery*. As noted in section 1, the terminology under analysis is not the terminology of the domain of middle-ear surgery, but the medical terminology used in one particular overview of this domain. Compared to the terminology of the domain, there may in principle be omissions due to the incompleteness of the overview or idiosyncrasies of the authors' language use. Much more significant, however, are the extensions beyond the specific domain, because there are many medical terms that are used to speak about middle-ear surgery without being themselves terms of that domain. Thus, Gersdorff & Gérard (2011: 10) give an overview of the layout of the operating room, including a drawing of how people and instruments should be arranged. In such a description, the terminology is from the domain of surgery in general, not specifically middle-ear surgery. At the same time, without such a description, the coverage of the domain would be incomplete.

In a first step, the sample of 747 terms was analysed morphologically. Less than 10% of the terms contain only one stem. Over 90% are compounds or phrases. Two-stem terms constitute more than half of the set, three-stem terms more than a quarter, which leaves only small portions of terms with four or five stems. Among two-stem terms, more than 90% can be analysed as compounds, the remainder as A+N phrases. For longer terms, the proportion of compounds seems, if anything, larger.

A remarkable feature of the set of terms is the almost complete absence of abbreviations. Among the five examples in our sample are the terms in (22).

(22) a. CSF leakage
b. CWU procedure

A first noteworthy property of (22) is that the abbreviations appear as non-heads of compounds. This is a general feature of all abbreviations in our sample. *CSF* in (22a) stands for *cerebrospinal fluid*. This is not a concept that is restricted to middle-ear surgery, but one that has a much more general medical application. *CWU* in (22b) stands for *canal wall up*. This and its antonym *canal wall down (CWD)* are the only abbreviations in our sample that are specific to the domain of middle-ear surgery. Gersdorff & Gérard 2011: 110) give the full form of *CWU* on introducing it for the first time and avoid using the abbreviation in titles and headings. Without a more extensive study of texts in the domain, it cannot be determined whether this is a general feature of the domain or an idiosyncratic feature of Gersdorff & Gérard (2011).

The dominance of compounds in the terminology in our sample makes the properties of compounding that affect transparency particularly relevant. In section 3, I identified three such properties:

- The relation between the head and the non-head of a compound is not made explicit in the form. If the head is derived from a verb, this verb tends to determine the relation.
- The internal structure is not visible in the form of the compound. This only applies for compounds with three or more stems.
- The non-head of a compound may be an identifier whose meaning does not contribute to the meaning of the whole compound.

Although the second and third of these properties only apply to a minority of the compounds in our sample, the general picture that arises is that most terms are not very transparent and that the frequent use of the word formation process of compounding is responsible.

However, an important factor in the evaluation of transparency has hardly been mentioned so far. A crucial factor for the interpretation of terms in general and compound terms in particular is knowledge of the specialized domain. Without domain knowledge, it is not possible to narrow down the set of possible relations to a set of plausible relations. In the solution of structural ambiguity, domain knowledge also indicates which combinations are plausible. In addition, however, domain knowledge also works at a more global level. A specialist in middle-ear surgery, or someone training to be one, will have a general picture of the field in which certain concepts are available. They will therefore not build up a hypothetical concept from scratch on the basis of various possible interpretations of a compound, but try to match the compound with a set of concepts they know. This is a much less complex task.

This alternative strategy explains why the problems in the interpretation of compounds are usually not perceived as strongly by domain specialists as they are by others. The most common group of users of texts with terminology apart from domain specialists is constituted by translators. The lack of transparency of compounds is therefore a much larger problem for translators than for domain specialists.

Acknowledgements

I would like to thank Franziska Steffan for her help with the manual extraction of terminology. When I use *we* or *our* for the sample, it is because of her share in collecting it. However, I am alone responsible for any errors in the analysis presented here.

References

Bauer, Laurie; Lieber, Rochelle & Plag, Ingo (2013), *The Oxford Reference Guide to English Morphology*, Oxford: Oxford University Press.

Corbeil, Jean-Claude & Archambault, Ariane (eds.) (1997), *Dictionnaire Visuel*, Paris: Fontaine.

Felek, Sevim Aslan; Celik, Hatice; Demirci, Munir; Islam, Ahmet; Elhan, Atilla H.; Samim, Erdal (2010), 'Type 2 ossiculoplasty: prognostic determination of hearing results by middle ear risk index', *American Journal of Otolaryngology* 31/5: 325-331.

Gersdorff, Michel & Gérard, Jean-Marc (2011), *Atlas of Middle Ear Surgery*, Stuttgart: Thieme.

ten Hacken, Pius (1994), *Defining Morphology: A Principled Approach to Determining the Boundaries of Compounding, Derivation, and Inflection*, Hildesheim: Olms.

—. (2003), 'Phrasal Elements as Parts of Words', in Hajičová, Eva; Kotěšovcová, Anna & Mírovský, Jiří (eds.), *Proceedings of CIL17*, CD-ROM, Praha: Matfyzpress, MFF UK.

—. (2012), 'Neoclassical word formation in English and the organization of the lexicon', in Gavriilidou, Zoe; Efthymiou, Angeliki; Thomadaki, Evangelia & Kambakis-Vougiouklis, Penelope (eds.), *Selected papers of the 10th International Conference of Greek Linguistics*, Komotini: Democritus University of Thrace, 78-88.

—. (2013), 'Compounds in English, in French, in Polish, and in General', *SKASE Journal of Theoretical Linguistics* 10: 97-113.

—. (2015a), 'Terms and Specialized Vocabulary: Taming the Prototypes', in Kockaert, Hendrik J. & Steurs, Frieda (eds.), *Handbook of Terminology: Volume 1*, Amsterdam: Benjamins, 3-13.

—. (2015b), 'Transposition and the Limits of Word Formation', in Bauer, Laurie; Körtvélyessy, Livia & Štekauer, Pavol (eds.), *Semantics of Complex Words*, Cham: Springer, pp. 187-216.

Jackendoff, Ray S. (1975), 'Morphological and Semantic Regularities in the Lexicon', *Language* 51: 639-671.

Levi, Judith N. (1978), *The syntax and semantics of complex nominals*, New York: Academic Press.

Marchand, Hans (1969), *The Categories and Types of Present-Day English Word-formation: A Synchronic-Diachronic Approach*, 2nd edition, München: Beck.

Roeper, Thomas & Siegel, Muffy (1978), 'A Lexical Transformation for Verbal Compounds', *Linguistic Inquiry* 9: 199-260.

Sadé, Jacob (1988), 'The four basic types of ossiculoplasty', in Babighian, Gregorio & Valdman, J.E. (eds.), *Transplants and Implants in Otology*, Amsterdam: Kugler & Ghedini Publications, 119.

Saussure, Ferdinand de (1916), *Cours de linguistique générale*, Charles Bally & Albert Sechehaye (eds.), Édition critique préparée par Tullio de Mauro, Paris: Payot, 1981.

CHAPTER FOUR

TRANSPARENCY AND USE OF NEOCLASSICAL WORD FORMATION IN MEDICAL ENGLISH

RENÁTA PANOCOVÁ

Medical English or English for Medical Purposes (EMP) has become prominent as the foremost international language of science and medicine (Ferguson, 2012). Research publications show a clear dominance of English, for instance Maher (1986) reports that in 1980 72.2% of the articles in the Index Medicus database were published in English. The role of national languages in medical research is decreasing. Giannoni (2008) finds out that more than 99% of medical journal papers by Italian authors are in English. Gunnarsson (2009) observes a similar tendency in Scandinavian countries.

The present situation contrasts with the middle ages when Latin was the dominant language in medicine. At that time, Latin was an international language not only in medicine, but also religion and philosophy (Fischbach, 1993: 94). In medicine, it remained influential in the 17th and even 18th century when essential medical works were in Latin, for example, *De Humani Corporis Fabrica* (1543) by the Belgian Andreas Vesalius (1514-1564), *Exercitatio de Motu Cordis et Sanguinis in Animalibus* (1628) by the Englishman William Harvey (1578-1657), or *Inventum Novum* (1761) by the Austrian Leopold Avenbrugger (1722-1809), (Fischbach, 1993: 94). Latin was universally understood among specialists. Despite the fact that Latin has been gradually replaced by English as a *lingua franca* in science, medical terminology today continues to be coined on the basis of Latin and Greek elements. These elements have been used in medicine for centuries and therefore it seems reasonable to hypothesize that there is a direct connection between universal understandability of Latin and Greek formatives and their semantic transparency in the terms used in a professional environment. This chapter explores degrees of semantic transparency of medical terms composed of

Latin and Greek items in comparison with eponyms, English equivalents and abbreviations or descriptive phrases.

The chapter is organized in five sections. Section 1 presents the notion of neoclassical word formation, describes its function in medical terminology and compares it with alternative naming strategies in the lexical field of diseases, syndromes, and symptoms. Section 2 discusses degrees of transparency of neoclassical names in contrast to eponyms. Section 3 analyses transparency of neoclassical names of diseases and their English equivalents. Section 4 concentrates on the analysis of semantic transparency of neoclassical terms and abbreviations and/or paraphrases. Section 5 summarizes the main findings and conclusions.

1 Neoclassical word formation in medical terminology

In general there is a correlation between a rapid progress in scientific development and new scientific terminology. The Oxford English Dictionary (OED) new words list from June 2014 includes such scientific terms as exemplified in (1).

(1) allobarbital, biopharma, biosimilar,
cholestasis, desalinize, ferrohydrodynamics,
heterodontosaurid, neonicotinoid, nutrigenetics,
nutrigenomics, trachodont, varioliform

A closer inspection reveals that scientific terms represent approximately one third out of the total number of 171 new entries in the June 2014 list. New words such as *biosimilar* ‘a biopharmaceutical drug designed to have active properties similar to one that has previously been licensed’, or *nutrigenomics* ‘the scientific study of the interaction of nutrition and genes, especially the role of diet in causing disease’, are obviously terms used in medical sciences. An interesting observation about these new entries is that they are formed by elements of Greek and Latin origin. Such formations are commonly referred to as neoclassical formations and they are frequent in medical terminology. It is obvious that the formations in (1) were not originally attested in Latin or Greek. They contrast with the examples of formations formed in Ancient Greek and Latin given in (2).

(2) a. astrology – ‘the practical application of the medieval art or science of astronomy’ (OED)
b. astronomy – ‘the science or art dealing with the positions and motions of planets and stars and their effect on natural phenomena and human affairs; in later use: the science

which deals with the universe beyond the earth's atmosphere, comprising the study of celestial objects and extraterrestrial phenomena, and of the nature and history of the universe' (OED)

In contrast to (1), the examples in (2) undoubtedly came into existence in ancient Greek and Latin. Interestingly, there is a semantic distinction between (2a) and (2b). According to OED (2015) Ancient Greek *ἀστρολογία* and *ἀστρονομία* were used interchangeably and both words denoted the science of celestial objects. Later, the Greeks of the Hellenistic period began to make calculations and predictions on the basis of astronomical observations, and the word *ἀστρολογία* came to be used in this sense. In Latin, *astrologia* appeared earlier (1st c. BCE) and predominantly in the sense of denoting the science of celestial objects. *Astronomia* first appeared a little later (in Seneca, 1st c. CE). In this chapter, neoclassical formations similar to (1) are the main subject of analysis.

Neoclassical formations constitute a substantial part of medical terminology; in general, anatomical terminology comes from Latin whereas most of the terms related to diagnosis and surgery have Greek origins (Willis, 2007: 1). Medical English or EMP includes medical terminology. Therefore it is useful to explore the relation between the essential notions of *word*, *concept* and *term*. The international standard defines the above-mentioned notions as follows in (3).

(3)
a. concept – 'unit of knowledge created by a unique combination of characteristics' (ISO 1087-1:2000)
b. term – 'verbal designation (3.4.1) of a general concept in a specific subject field' (ISO 1087-1:2000)
c. word – 'smallest linguistic unit conveying a specific meaning and capable of existing as a separate unit in a sentence' (ISO 5127:2001)

The definition of the object in (3a) indicates that it belongs to the field of cognitive science. In (3b) and (3c), it is obvious that objects are from the study of language where the former is a unit of terminology and the latter of linguistics. The relationship between (3a) and (3b) may be expressed by the equation concept = content, term = form (Masár, 1991). This means that (3a) and (3b) are united and the leading or superordinate element is (3a). (3b) is a way of representation of (3a). If content and form are the categories of one object, a question about the nature of object arises. The object is a term with two dimensions; a set of properties characterizing content and a set of formal constituents (morphemes) i.e. form. Bodnár

(1982) claims that in a systemic approach, the interpretation of the relationship between (3a) and (3b) is based on two assumptions. First, the whole (system) has specific properties that may be different from the properties of individual components. Second, a system is governed by its own rules, and these rules cannot be derived from the rules which govern the behaviour of its components. A term always represents a particular concept or a type of concepts and there is a direct link between them. In contrast, the relationship between a term and an object is indirect because it requires mental activity of our brain to evoke an image of the object. For instance, from the perspective of terminology, *laryngoscope* 'an apparatus which by a combination of mirrors enables an observer to inspect a patient's larynx' (OED, 2015), is an existing physical object, or an instrument used for medical examination and it corresponds to (3b). The idea of *laryngoscope* created in our mind when we encounter the instrument is referred to by (3a). OED (2015) gives (4) as an example for *laryngoscope* in the sense of (3c)

(4) There is no trace of a laryngoscope before the middle of the eighteenth century.[1]

In (4), *laryngoscope* is a linguistic unit functioning as a noun in the sense of (3c). At the same time it is a linguistic sign having a form and a meaning.

In a semiotic perspective, a term is a special type of a lexical sign (Furdík, 2008: 62). Furdík (2008: 63) makes a distinction between the semiotic structure of a term and a non-term as illustrated in Figure 4-1.

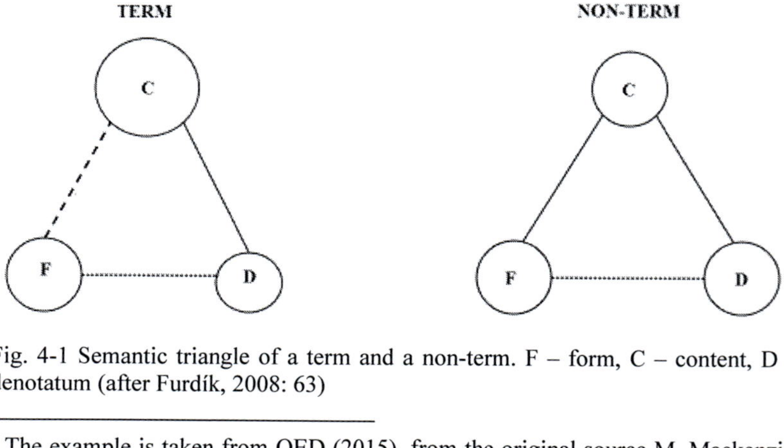

Fig. 4-1 Semantic triangle of a term and a non-term. F – form, C – content, D - denotatum (after Furdík, 2008: 63)

[1] The example is taken from OED (2015), from the original source M. Mackenzie (1880) *Man. Dis. Throat & Nose* I. 213

Figure 4-1 shows that the content of a term is placed in a larger circle. This means it is semantically richer than the content of a non-term. A term has more properties than a general lexical item, for example, the term *water* is defined as 'H_2O; a clear, odourless, tasteless liquid, solidifying at 32°F (0°C and R) and boiling at 212°F (100°C, 80°R) that is present in all animal and vegetable tissues and dissolves more substances than any other liquid' is characterized by more semantic properties than a commonly used non-term *water* 'the clear liquid that falls as rain and is used for things such as drinking and washing' (Furdík, 2008: 62). Another difference between a term and non-term in Figure 4-1 is in the connection between content and form. The connection is weaker in a term as opposed to a non-term. This is represented by a dotted line in Figure 4-1. It is exemplified in (5).

(5) a. atomic power
    b. nuclear power

The examples in (5) illustrate that when human knowledge advances, it is possible to replace the old designator (form) by a new one denoting the same concept. The term in (5a) was attested in 1824 (OED, 2015) and is obsolete at present. Scientific research revealed that power does not originate from the atom as a whole, but from its nucleus. This means that onomasiologically, (5b) more accurately denotes the concept. According to OED (2015), the term in (5b) was first attested more than a hundred years later than (5a) in 1945.

In contrast to Furdík's (2008) semiotic basis Horecký (1982) approaches terminology from an onomasiological perspective. He defines *term* as a four-dimensional object with four components: conceptual, semantic, onomasiological, and onomatological. An overview of these components is given in Table 4-1.

Table 4-1 starts from the conceptual component of term. It includes a set of logical predicates, a logical spectrum of a concept, or in other words, simple sentences describing its characteristic properties. Table 4-1 exemplifies the conceptual component with a medical term *retractor* 'any of numerous devices (now usually metal instruments of different shapes and sizes) used to hold open an incision or orifice, or to hold structures away from the field of operation' (OED, 2015).

Components of term	**Content**	**Example** ***retractor***
conceptual	predicates	It is inanimate substance. The inanimate substance is material and made of metal. It is designed for performing an action, etc.
semantic	semantic features	Instrument, to draw or pull (a thing) back
onomasiological	motives	Onomasiological base: Agent Onomasiological mark (derivational base): Action
onomatological	morphemes	Action => *retract* Agent => *-or*

Table 4-1 Four components of term

The semantic component of a term specifies semantic features of a concept. The semantic features are selected from the set of the abstracted properties based on logical predicates of a concept. They are expressed by words and morphemes. In our example *retractor*, the semantic feature ‘designed for performing an action’ is represented by the constituent *retract* ‘to draw or pull (a thing) back’. The semantic feature ‘a tool from a class of instruments’ is expressed by the derivational morpheme *-or*. The form of the semantic component is determined by the order of semantic features expressed in the conceptual component. A semantic feature can be assigned to any predicate from the conceptual component. In the example *retractor*, two semantic features were selected to be represented by morphemes.

The onomasiological component of a term explains a degree of motivation of the selected semantic features in a naming unit. This component explains the connection between meaning and word formation constituents. The onomasiological component consists of a form and content. The content is represented by selected semantic features which explain the motivation of a term. The form specifies the relationship between the onomasiological base and the onomasiological mark. The onomasiological base in the example *retractor* is the suffix *-or*. It is modified by the onomasiological mark or derivational base *retract*. These reflect the meaning ‘an instrument for drawing or pulling (a thing) back’. In a multi-word term, e.g. *mammary gland*, the noun *gland* represents the onomasiological base and is modified by the onomasiological mark represented by the adjective *mammary*.

The onomatological component of a term is a linguistic representation of its individual constituents. This component is language-specific whereas the conceptual component is universal. In *retractor*, the derivational suffix -*or* is specified by the action the verb *retract* denotes.

Terms are characterized by their specific properties: precision, unambiguity, semantic transparency, systematism, derivability (Furdík, 2008: 61). These features are in line, for instance, with Wright (2006: 29), who highlights transparency, consistency, appropriateness, economy (conciseness), derivability, linguistic correctness and local language policy with respect to the use of "native language" term elements as general principles for term formation. Gilreath (1995) views transparency as the most essential of his sixteen criteria to be applied in resolving terminological disputes. He defines transparency as "the degree to which a term's elements immediately signify its intended meaning; for a transparent term, one can see the meaning in its morphology (assuming one knows the meanings of the term elements" (Gilreath, 1995: 34). He distinguishes four types of transparency: semantic, code, typographic and phonetic, and considers semantic transparency the most relevant. Interestingly, he differentiates between semantic transparency and the precision of terms. Gilreath (1995: 34) claims that precise terms may not necessarily be transparent, for instance, the term *Johnson effect* 'heat effect' is precise, but non-transparent.

Horecký (1956, 1967), Masár (1991), and Furdík (2008) do not make a principled distinction between semantic transparency and motivation, although there has been some development in the use of these terms. Horecký (1956) uses the term *významová priezračnosť* 'semantic transparency', Masár (1991) *motivovanosť* 'motivatedness', and Furdík (2008) equates the notions *významová priezračnosť* 'semantic transparency', *slovotvorná motivovanosť* 'word formation motivatedness', and *existencia onomaziologickej štruktúry* 'the existence of an onomasiological structure'.

Let us now turn to exploring how these notions are linked to Saussure's *arbitrariness* of the linguistic sign. According to Saussure, there is no direct connection between the *signifier* (form) and the *signified* (meaning). This is exemplified by the existence of different names in different languages for the same concept, e.g. *lungs* in English, *pľúca* in Slovak, or *poumons* in French. Furdík (2008: 30) emphasizes that from a semasiological perspective it is possible to accept that the sequence of sounds /lʌŋz/ is not in a causal relationship with the body organ it denotes.

This means it does not answer the question 'What are lungs?'. From this perspective, the notion of *arbitrariness* is valid for each linguistic sign viewed only in isolation (Dolník, 1990: 148) including complex or derived words. In contrast, when we ask 'What is muscularity?', the word formation structure gives us not the answer, but a hint of relevant information about the denotatum, e.g. 'a condition related to muscles'. This naturally presupposes understanding of the base word *muscle*. For Dolník (1990) and Furdík (2008), this moment is a turning point from viewing a word in isolation to seeing it in relation with other lexical items. Furdík (2008: 31) claims that a lexical item is not arbitrary, but motivated. His understanding of motivation is that we can explain why a concept has a particular name. Motivation does not play a role when taking into account a lexical item in isolation. Furdík (2008: 31) illustrates this difference with the example *cow*. In his view, Saussure took into account an isolated lexeme *cow*, but did not take into account that *cow* is named *cow* because it differs from *bull*. According to (Furdík, 2008: 31) this means that each differentiated lexical item must be motivated because differentation is the basis for a causal relationship between the form and the content. Arbitrariness is valid only for an isolated item and from the semasiological perspective (Furdík, 2008: 32). On the basis of two key assumptions, non-isolation of a lexeme and onomasiological approach, Furdík (2008: 32) views the lexicon as an organised system of a set of lexemes connected by a web of basic and superstructural *lexical motivations*. Furdík (2008: 32) claims that *motivation* is the most important principle of the organisation of the lexis. The sum of all types of motivation contributes to the fact that the lexeme is an individual unit. For Furdík (2008) *lexical motivation* is an inherent property of all lexemes included in the lexis of a language. Lexical motivaton is viewed as a possibility to answer the question 'Why is X named like this?' synchronically and as a property or as a web of relations among lexical items. Furdík distinguishes several types of *lexical motivation*, including word formation, terminological and abbreviating motivation. The results of the research by Furdík (1990) demonstrate that motivated lexical items in Slovak clearly dominate, with the ratio of 65% motivated lexical items to 35% unmotivated lexical items.

In this context, it is interesting to remark that in terminology Furdík (2008: 62) admits a greater degree of arbitrariness (cf. the example in (5) and Figure 4-1). Researchers frequently struggle with the search for the best term to name one and the same concept. This means that the relationship between two designators is less limited and researchers take responsibility. The greater freedom in naming for researchers is given with respect to a degree of arbitrariness (Furdík, 2008: 62).

It is not surprising that in an onomasiological perspective the role of motivation is immediately obvious. This raises a question about the relationship between motivation and transparency. Furdík (2008) does not distinguish motivation and transparency as mentioned above. In his onomasiological theory of word formation, Štekauer (to appear) views semantic transparency as listener/reader friendly in contrast to economy of expression, which is speaker/writer friendly. He does not discuss motivation. Although there may be a certain degree of overlap between motivation and transparency, the communicative perspective may serve as a basis for the distinction between the two notions. If transparency is linked to the listener/reader perspective, then motivation is closer to the speaker/writer perspective. The role of a speaker in the name-finding process is dominant in onomasiological approaches. The new name, however, must be accepted by a speech community representing the listener/reader perspective. This means that both terms may be distinct in certain contexts though both are compatible in their use in word formation. This is in line with ten Hacken (this volume), who also relates motivation to the speaker choosing a name and transparency to the hearer interpreting the name. In this paper, I will use the term transparency in line with Horecký's (1956), Masár's (1991) and Furdík's (2008) definition of motivation in terminology.

As indicated above, neoclassical word formation is used extensively in medical terminology. Below, I will examine the transparency of this naming device in comparison to alternative naming strategies, such as English variants and eponyms. Medical terms denoting syndromes, symptoms, and diseases were collected from Stedman's (1997) medical dictionary. Then the terms were divided into three categories. The first class covers neoclassical medical terms with an English equivalent. The second category is represented by neoclassical medical terms with synonymous eponyms. The last class includes neoclassical medical terms with abbreviations and/or paraphrases.

2 Neoclassical word formation versus eponyms

Eponyms frequently occur in medical terminology. Although eponyms were for the first time excluded from the official Latin anatomical nomenclature *Parisiensia Nomina Anatomica* (PNA) in 1955, they are still popular among medical specialists because they are concise and precise (Musil et al., 2010: 61). Eponyms might be preferred in cases when it is difficult to determine one or two characteristic properties of the concept they name, which could be then used in their formal structure. It is therefore not surprising that eponyms are often used in naming diseases, syndromes and symptoms. Poláčková (1992: 345) claims that one of the possible reasons for their popularity among specialists may be their low degree of transparency and intelligibility to laymen. This may play a role in medical confidentiality. In anatomical nomenclature, there is no reason to make a term less intelligible to the general public. This may explain the gradual replacement of eponyms in anatomical terminology by more transparent terms as indicated in (6).

(6) Achilles tendon → tendo calcaneus, heel tendon
Bartholin's gland → greater vestibular gland
Corti's organ → spiral organ
Hesselbach's triangle → inguinal triangle
Wirsung's canal→ pancreatic duct

The eponyms in (6) illustrate that eponyms do not provide transparent information about their meaning. Caspar Bartholin the Younger (1655-1738), Alfonso Corti (1822-1876), Franz Kaspar Hesselbach (1759–1816), and Johann Georg Wirsung (1589-1643) were anatomists who discovered the anatomical structures described by the second constituents in (5). Given the fact that the anatomists lived between 16th and 19th centuries, it may be assumed that eponyms have become lexicalized and the names may be familiar only to specialists in the history of human anatomy who have more detailed knowledge about etymology. This contrasts with *Achilles tendon* being named after the Greek mythological character. Here it may be hypothesized that the eponym may be more transparent to the general public, at least in European cultures. This example illustrates that transparency is a matter of degree rather than an absolute notion. The examples in (7) compare degrees of transparency of medical eponyms with their neoclassical equivalents.

(7) a. Bannister's disease = angioedema
b. Cruveilier's disease = amyotrophic lateral sclerosis
c. Busse-Buschke disease = cryptococcosis
d. Swift's disease = acrodynia

In (7a), the eponym *Bannister's disease* seems non-transparent as its meaning 'recurrent large circumscribed areas of subcutaneous edema of sudden onset, usually disappearing within 24 hours'[2] cannot be interpreted on the basis of its constituents. Its neoclassical synonym *angioedema* seems semantically more transparent, providing that a hearer is familiar with the meaning of the individual neoclassical formatives *angio-* 'blood or lympth vessels' and *edema* 'a swelling; an accumulation of an excessive amount of watery fluid in cells, tissues, or serous cavities'. Gilreath (1995: 35) lists several subjective aspects of transparency, such as "different connotation of words and word elements and different levels of familiarity with those term elements", and these must be taken into account for the whole language community. Despite an inevitable component of subjectivity, Gilreath (1995: 35) claims "there is a degree of objectivity in rating this criterion". Evaluating the degree of transparency of *Bannister's disease* and the neoclassical formation *angioedema* in (7a) is clearly in favour of the latter, especially among medical specialists. All medical professionals are trained in acquiring the meaning of prefixes, suffixes, and combining forms of Latin and Greek origin commonly used in medical terminology. Therefore it seems reasonable to assume that less extra time is required to interpret the meaning of the neoclassical term. The eponym may be more transparent to a narrow group of medical professionals who encounter the term frequently, but less transparent to specialists working in other domains.

From an onomasiological perspective, the preference for terms with a transparent mapping of conceptual structure onto onomasiological structure represented by word formation constituents or formatives is one of the key properties of terms (Horecký, 1956, 1982; Masár, 1991; Furdík 2008, etc.). The four-dimensional model of the term by Horecký (1982), explaining conceptual and onomasiological structure, was presented in Table 4-1 above. Sets of relationships among constituents in the lexis may be regarded as an indicator of transparency of terms. It is exemplified in (8).

(8) a. angio- → angiography → angiographic → angiographically
edema → edematize → edematization

b.

angio-	edema
angioblast	cerebral edema
angiology	pulmonary edema
angiodysplasia	
angiogenic	
angiopoiesis	

[2] Unless otherwise indicated all definitions are taken from Stedman (1997).

Furdík (2008: 49) labels a set of constituents such as (8a) a word formation line. It is the order of motivated items where a subsequent item is formed on the basis of the preceding one. The element *angio-* combines with *-graphy* to form the output meaning 'radiography of vessels after the injection of a radiopaque contrast material'. This is the base for the derivation of *angiographic* 'relating to or utilizing angiography', which gives rise to the formation of *angiographically* 'by means of angiography'. A similar word formation line is given for *edema*. The instances in (8b) illustrate Furdík's notion of a word formation paradigm defined as an organized set of complex words formed on the basis of the same motivating element. The complex words are not derived from each other. For example, *angioblast* means 'a cell taking part in blood vessel formation' and *angiodysplasia* is 'degenerative or congenital structural abnormality of the normally distributed vasculature'. Both terms are clearly related to blood vessels, but the latter is not directly derived from the former or vice versa. Similarly, *cerebral edema* plays no role in forming *pulmonary edema*. Each term denotes a different type of *edema*. Word formation lines and word formation paradigms may combine, for instance, resulting in *angioedema*. A set of word formation lines and word formation paradigms derived from one unmotivated or underived item is labelled word formation nest (Furdík, 2008: 49). The eponym *Bannister's disease* obviously does not enter into relations of the type in (8). The formal structure is easy to determine, but the meaning cannot be straightforwardly identified, it is closer to non-transparent.

In (7b), the neoclassical variant *amyotrophic lateral sclerosis* is longer than the corresponding eponym *Cruveilier's disease*. However, the interpretability of 'a disease of motor tracts of the lateral columns and anterior horns of the spinal cord, causing progressive muscular atrophy, increased reflexes, fibrillary twitching and spastic irritability of muscles' is straightforward and it is fully compositional. *Amyotrophic* means 'related to muscular atrophy', *lateral* 'on the side', and *sclerosis* 'hardening of tissue'. The length of the neoclassical term does not conform to the principle of economy, which may be a reason for the use of the abbreviation *ALS*. Stedman (1997) lists it together with the dictionary entry, but does not include it in a separate list of common medical abbreviations. Although the abbreviated form reduces transparency, it still seems more transparent than the eponym. Stedman (1997) gives five different eponyms denoting *amyotrophic lateral sclerosis* presented in alphabetical order in (9).

(9) a. Aran-Duchenne disease = amyotrophic lateral sclerosis
b. Duchenne-Aran disease = amyotrophic lateral sclerosis

c. Charcot's disease = amyotrophic lateral sclerosis
d. Cruveilier's disease = amyotrophic lateral sclerosis
e. Lou Gehring's disease = amyotrophic lateral sclerosis

The reversed order of the names in (9a) and (9b) is common in medical eponyms. The use is customary. It may also be determined culturally and regionally. In Europe, the eponyms (9a), (9b) and (9c) are widespread. F.A. Aran and G.B. Duchenne de Boulogne are credited with a clinical description around 1850 (Eisen & Kriegen, 2006: 27). Jean Martin Charcot was a recognized French neurologist who described this disease not only clinically, but also pathologically in 1869 (Galalaldeen & Hart, 2007: 327). In the USA, the eponym (7e) is frequent. It is in memory of the famous baseball player Lou Gehring who died of the disease (Galalaldeen & Hart2007: 327). Interestingly, the *International Statistical Classification of Diseases and Related Health Problems 10th Revision* (ICD-10) Version for 2010 lists the neoclassical term without mentioning any of the eponyms in (9) in brackets although it is a common practice with many other diseases. An online search, however, relates the eponyms in (9a) and (9b) to *amyotrophic lateral sclerosis*. The remaining ones do not give any search results.

It is interesting to observe that the abbreviation ALS enters into a word formation line and a word formation paradigm. A Google search gives the formations in (10).

(10) a. ALS → ALS patient → ALS patient stories
b. ALS
ALS patient
ALS fact sheet
ALS symptom
ALS expert
ALS society

In general, the meaning of abbreviations is determined by the meaning of the unabbreviated form. Abbreviations represent a specific type of lexemes and they gradually may become part of the language system (Furdík, 2008: 71). The word formation line and word formation paradigm in (10) may be seen as evidence. The word formation line in (10a) starts with the abbreviation *ALS*, which becomes a basis for *ALS patient*, which recurs in *ALS patient stories*. The word formation paradigm in (10b) includes a list of items related by the abbreviation, but not derived directly from each other.

Returning to the examples of eponyms in (7), in (7c) the degree of transparency of the neoclassical term *cryptococcosis* is weaker. The main reason is a different analysis of individual constituents of the neoclassical term. Although *Cryptococcus* is formed by *crypto-* 'hidden, obscure' and *coccus* 'berry', its meaning is 'a genus of yeastlike fungi that reproduces by budding'. The element *-osis* denotes 'process, condition, state'. The meaning of *cryptococcosis* is 'infection by *Cryptococcus neoformans*, causing a pulmonary, disseminated, or meningeal mycosis'. The eponym *Busse-Buschke disease* is non-transparent and relatively difficult to pronounce, which reduces the degree of conciseness (economy). Similar to the examples in (9a) and (9b), an online search in the international classification of diseases relates the eponym *Busske-Buschke* disease to *cryptococcosis* without direct reference in the classification.

In (7d) the example of the eponym *Swift's disease* and the synonymous neoclassical term *acrodynia* is presented. The latter seems interesting from the perspective of evaluating the degree of semantic transparency. The meaning of the constituent formative *acro-* is 'extreme, topmost, outermost' and *-dynia* 'pain'. The semantically transparent meaning of *acrodynia* is then 'pain in peripheral or acral parts of the body'. The situation is more complex, because the term *acrodynia* has another sense. It is only this second sense 'a syndrome caused almost exclusively by mercury poisoning: in children, characterized by erythrema of the extremities, chest, and nose, polyneuritis, and gastrointestinal symptoms; in adults, by anorexia, photophobia, sweating and tachycardia' that is synonymous to *Swift's disease*. The degree of transparency in the second sense of *acrodynia* largely disappears because the meaning cannot be identified on the basis of the meaning of constituent parts of the term. Stedman (1997) also gives the English synonym *pink disease*. The English equivalent seems slightly more semantically transparent than the neoclassical term. The eponym *Swift's disease* is further on the scale towards non-transparency.

3 Neoclassical word formation versus English terms

A number of neoclassical names of diseases have equivalent English terms. The English terms are often multi-word expressions and are listed in the ICD (2010). Some examples are given in (11).

(11) a. osteoarthritis = degenerative joint disease
b. otitis externa = swimmer's ear

c. erythroblastosis fetalis = ABO hemolytic disease of the newborn
d. erythrema infectiosum = fifth disease

The examples in (11) demonstrate that, especially in terminology, multi-word units are common. Furdík (2008: 50) defines multi-word units as lexical units that can be labelled as a syntagm; their form is larger than one content word, but they name the phenomena that are perceived by a speech community as units. In some cases, a single-word naming unit cannot express the required number of semantic features of a particular denotatum. Furdík (2008: 50) points to the fact that languages solve such borderline issues in various ways: For instance, German, Finnish, or Turkish prefer complex words resulting from the word formation process of compounding. A similar tendency is observed in English or Chinese. By contrast, in Slovak or Russian, compounding is used less and multi-word units represent an alternative type of naming (for more details cf. Furdík, 2008: 50-53).

The neoclassical formation in (11a) is composed of the elements *osteo-* 'bone', *arthr-* 'joint' and *-itis* 'inflammation' and Stedman (1997) gives as meaning of the name 'arthritis characterized by erosion of articular cartilage, which becomes soft, frayed, and thinned with eburnation of subchondral bone and outgrowths of marginal osteophytes'. The English equivalent gives us similarly relevant information. The advantage of the English term is its high degree of transparency, the meaning can easily be interpreted not only by a specialist, but also by a layman. The neoclassical equivalent is transparent to a similar degree to an expert in the field or to a non-expert with a sufficient knowledge of Latin and Greek. The disadvantage of the English equivalent is its length, which violates the economy principle.

In (11b) the neoclassical term is composed of two independent words *otitis* 'inflammation of the ear' and *externa* 'outside'. The former is complex with the two elements *ot-* 'ear' and *-itis* 'inflammation'. The meaning of the neoclassical name is transparent; its meaning can be deduced from the meaning of its constituents. The English counterpart is not a calque of the neoclassical term. It clearly highlights a different semantic feature of this condition. It immediately provides the information that this type of infection 'often develops in persons who swim frequently and get water trapped in their ears' (Stedman, 1997). Onomasiologically, both terms are transparent, but they differ in the selection of semantic properties reflected in the onomasiological component and the onomatological component of the two terms. The four-dimensional description of the terms in line with Horecký (1982) is presented in Table 4-2.

Components of term	**Term** *otitis externa*	**Term** *swimmer's ear*
conceptual	It is a process. It causes discomfort. It affects body parts, etc.	It is a process. It causes discomfort. It affects body parts. Its presence is caused by water, etc.
semantic	Process of inflammation affecting the ear	Process of infection affecting the ear, typical for people who often swim
onomasiological	Onomasiological base: Process Onomasiological mark: Location	Onomasiological base: Theme Onomasiological mark: Quality
onomatological	Location => *externa* Process => *otitis*	Quality => *swimmer's* Theme => *ear*

Table 4-2 Four components of the terms *otitis externa* and *swimmer's ear*

The comparison of the onomasiological structure of both terms reveals interesting similarities and differences. Conceptual components of the terms share the spectrum of logical predicates. Semantic features are similar although the English counterpart includes the property 'typical for people who often swim'. The fact that this property is selected here is essential because it is mapped onto the morphological structure of *swimmer's ear*. The body part which is affected is represented by *ear*. This means that the English term emphasizes the body part affected by the condition and modifies who is likely to be influenced. In the neoclassical term, the process of inflammation is represented by a neoclassical formative *-itis* and the place of the Process is specified by the onomasiological mark *ot-* 'ear', and it is modified by *externa* emphasizing it is influenced by the outside factors.

Returning to our examples in (11), (11c) represents an interesting case to discuss. The meaning of the neoclassical term is 'a grave hemolytic anemia that, in most instances, results from the development in the mother of anti-Rh antibody in response to the Rh factor in the (Rh-positive) fetal blood; it is characterized by many erythroblasts in the circulation' (Stedman, 1997). The meaning is transparent and based on the meaning of *erythroblastosis* 'the presence of erythroblasts in considerable number in the blood' while *erythroblast* is 'the first generation of cells in the red blood cells series that can be distinguished from precursor endothelial cells' and *-osis* 'condition'. *Fetalis* pertains to the newborn. The literal meaning does not include any information about the cause of this condition, the Rh-factor. This contrasts with the English descriptive phrase *ABO hemolytic disease of the newborn*. The first element *ABO* refers to a blood group, *hemolytic* means 'destructive to blood cells' *disease* explains the condition deviates from normal and *of the newborn* specifies in which type of patients the condition occurrs. The English counterpart is semantically richer; it covers more characteristic properties of the condition than the neoclassical one. On the other hand, it includes a neoclassical element, *hemolytic*, which requires extra knowledge to decode its meaning. At the same time, the English term is not concise, it is the longest one among all examples in (11).

In (11d), the names of the disease show a contrast between a relatively high transparency of the neoclassical term and much reduced transparency of the English synonym. *Erythrema* is 'redness of the skin due to capillary dilatation', and *infectiosum* explains it is caused by infection. *Fifth disease* is precise and concise, but the correct interpretation requires the background knowledge that the *first*, *second*, *third*, *fourth* and *fifth diseases* all denote common childhood illnesses characterized by a rash.

It has been hypothesized that there is a correlation between semantic transparency and frequency of N+N compounds in English (Bell and Schäfer, 2015). In the light of their findings, it is interesting to search for easily accessible frequency data via Google. Although Google figures are not always reliable and a brief scanning of the results shows that both terms may be used in the same hit, the proportions in most cases are clear enough to draw at least a tentative conclusion.[3] An overview of the results is in Table 4-3.

Neoclassical term	*Google hits*	*English term*	*Google hits*
osteoarthrosis	14700	degenerative joint disease	2060
otitis externa	1290	swimmer's ear	744
erythroblastosis fetalis	95	ABO hemolytic disease of the newborn	95,6
erythrema infectiosum	129	fifth disease	5470

Table 4-3 Google hits (in thousands) for neoclassical terms and their English equivalents

Table 4-3 shows that the most striking difference in the number of hits is in the occurrence of *erythrema infectiosum* versus *fifth disease* in favour of the latter. In contrast, the neoclassical term *osteorarhtrosis* was found seven times more often than its English counterpart *degenerative joint disease*. The English term is not concise enough, which may play a role in its frequency. It is interesting to see the results for *erythroblastosis fetalis* versus *ABO hemolytic disease of the newborn*. The Google hits are approximately the same, less than 1% higher for the English counterpart.

4 Neoclassical word formation versus abbreviations

Abbreviations may be defined as phonetic and orthographic units that function as words or naming units (Furdík, 2008: 70). The process of abbreviating is in line with the economy principle in language and it has been part of linguistic communication since ancient times. Pictographic writing may be considered as one example of abbreviating. A pictogram may represent a whole statement. Abbreviation in its linguistic sense appeared after the invention of phonetically inspired writing. This type of

[3] Google figures were retrieved on 24 May, 2015.

writing is characterized by its spatial linearity, which corresponds to some degree with temporal linearity. Furdík (2008: 70) points to the fact that spatial linearity of writing requires more time than temporal linearity of speaking or spoken language and this explains the presence of abbrevations in old written documents, for instance *SPQR* = *Senatus Popolusque Romanus* 'The Senate and People of Rome', or *INRI* = *Iesus Nazarenus Rex Iudaeorum* 'Jesus the Nazarene, King of the Jews'. The written documents from the middle ages include precise lists of abbreviations used in manuscripts in the codex format (Furdík, 2008: 70).

Basic properties of abbreviations are the tendency to include the smallest possible number of relevant elements while preserving communicative efficiency of the resulting output. The understanding of the meaning of abbreviations is determined by the understanding of the meaning of the unabbreviated input; abbreviations are mnemonic. The use of many abbreviations may be temporally limited and their inventory reflects social phenomena relevant at a specific time.

Abbreviations are frequent in medical language and many specialized dictionaries include a separate section with common medical abbreviations, e.g. Stedman (1997). It is interesting to observe that also some neoclassical names of diseases are abbreviated. This is illustrated in (12).

(12) a. adrenoleukodystrophy = ALD
b. acute necrotizing ulcerative gingivitis = ANUG
c. hereditary erythroblastic multinuclearity associated with positive acidified serum = HEMPAS

The example in (12a) demonstrates the need to economize extremely complex terms. The neoclassical name is precise, denoting 'an inherited (X-linked recessive) disorder characterized by atrophy of the adrenal cortex and degeneration of the white matter of the nervous system, typically appearing in prepubertal boys' (OED, 2015). The name is transparent and its meaning can be deduced on the basis of the meanings of its constituents, *adreno-* 'relating to the adrenal gland', *leuko-* 'white, white blood cells', *dystrophy* 'progressive changes that may result from defective nutrition of a tissue or organ', this element is complex, composed of *dys-* 'bad, difficult' and *-trophy* 'food, nutrition'. The abbreviated form makes use of the first letters of the three main constituents; it is an example of an initialism. It is interesting that Stedman (1997) lists the abbreviation in (12a) in the section on common medical abbreviations, but the neoclassical term is not listed in the dictionary. The abbreviation *ALD* is included in the main part of the Stedman dictionary, but it represents 'assistive listening device', a completely different concept. This ambiguity as to the full form further reduces the degree of transparency of the (12a) abbreviation as opposed to the full neoclassical term.

The example in (12b) illustrates a long multi-word medical term containing complex elements. It contrasts with the single-word item in (12a). The abbreviation in (12b) is an acronym and it may be pronounced as one word. The full form is transparent and precise because it captures all important characteristics of the condition. It is obvious that it is a type of *gingivitis* 'inflammation of the gingiva as a response to bacterial plaque on adjacent teeth'. Another characteristic feature is the presence of ulcers and *necrosis* 'pathologic death of one or more cells, or of a portion of tissue or organ'. Many diseases can appear in its acute or chronic form, which explains the relevance of this information. The main disadvantage of the full form is its length. The abbreviation in (12b) is relatively easy to pronounce and remember. Stedman (1997) also gives an English counterpart of (12b), *trench mouth*. Although it is concise when compared to its neoclassical variant, it seems less transparent. The English term is metaphorical and the correct interpretation requires the information that the condition was frequent among soldiers in the First World War.

In (12c), an example of an extremely long and complex term is given. It can also be seen that there might be a correlation between the length of the multi-word term and the length of the corresponding abbreviation. The abbreviated form in (12c) is the longest one in (12). It is an acronym pronounced as a word. Similar to (12a), Stedman (1997) includes the abbreviation and its full form in (12c) in the section on common medical abbreviations, but neither of them is listed in the main dictionary part.

What the examples in (12) illustrate is that abbreviations are mnemonic and very economic in expression, but much less transparent than neoclassical formations. They are motivated, but the hearer or reader will have to reconstruct this motivation on the basis of knowledge of the concepts in a field. A further problem for transparency is the frequent ambiguity of abbreviated forms.

5 Conclusion: The relative transparency of neoclassical word formation

The aim of the analysis in this chapter was to examine semantic transparency of neoclassical word formation and compare it with that of eponyms, English counterparts of the names of diseases and abbreviations. The results can be illustrated by the continuum in Figure 4-2.

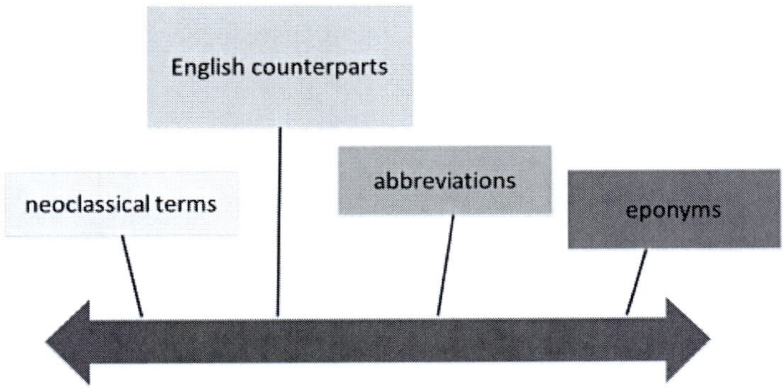

Fig. 4-2 Degrees of transparency of medical terms

The double arrow in Figure 4-2 points to the fact that semantic transparency is a matter of degree; it is scalar. The left-hand end of the arrow represents full transparency whereas the extreme right is entirely opaque. There is no scale on the continuum, because there is no obvious way to assign a numeric value to a degree of transparency. However, individual expressions and classes of expressions can be represented relatively to each other.

Neoclassical names of diseases display a greater semantic transparency than their eponymous synonyms. The degree of transparency may vary depending on two important factors: the polysemy of neoclassical formatives and their economy of expression. For instance, the examples (7b) and (7d) illustrate how an increase in these two factors reduces transparency. The comparison of neoclassical terms and their English counterparts shows that the degree of transparency may be influenced by the selection of semantic features represented by neoclassical formatives and English constituents. Although not all neoclassical terms will be to the left of all English terms, there is a clear tendency for the former to be more transparent. The comparison of neoclassical names of diseases and their abbreviations clearly demonstrates a greater degree of transparency of the former. The abbreviations are mnemonic and their correct understanding depends on the knowledge of the full term. Different degrees of transparency can be observed not only relative to eponyms, English equivalents and abbreviations, but also internally within each class. The factors influencing the degree of semantic transparency are the same, economy and polysemy. It can be concluded that neoclassical word formation is a relatively efficient naming device in the sense that it strikes a good balance between conciseness and transparency, as long as the names are mainly used by specialists.

References

Bell, Melanie J. & Schäfer, Martin (2015), 'Modelling semantic transparency in English compound nouns.', in Pirrelli, Vito; Marzi, Claudia; Ferro, Marcello (eds.), *Word Structure and Word Usage, Proceedings of the NetWordS Final Conference, Pisa, March 30-April 1, 2015*, published at http://ceur-ws.org, 63-65.

Bodnár, Ján (1982), 'Nová idea systémovosti.' [New idea of systemicity], *Nedělná Pravda*, 19. 2. 1982: 6.

Dolník, Juraj (1990), *Lexikálna sémantika* [Lexical semantics], Bratislava: Univerzita Komenského.

Eisen, Andrew & Kriegen, Charles (2006), *Amyotrophic Lateral Sclerosis. A Synthesis of Research and Clinical Practice*, Cambridge: Cambridge University Press.

Ferguson, Gibson (2012), 'English for Medical Purposes.', in Paltridge, Brian and Starfield, Sue (eds.), *The Handbook of English for Specific Purposes*, Oxford: Wiley-Blackwell, pp. 243-262.

Fischbach, Henry (1993), 'Translation, the Great Pollinator of Science', in Wright, Sue Ellen & Wright Jr., Leland D. (eds.), *Scientific and Technical Translation*, Amsterdam/Philadelphia: John Benjamins, 89-100.

Furdík, Juraj (1990), 'Pokus o komplexný kvantitatívny výskum slovotvorného systému pomocou počítača. (Metodologické východiská a prvé výsledky.)' [An attempt on complex computer-based quantitative research into the word formation system. (Methodological assumptions and initial results)], in Blanár, Vincent (ed.), *Metódy výskumu a opisu lexiky slovanských jazykov. Materiály zo sympózia konaného v rámci 7. zasadnutia Lexikologicko- -lexikografickej komisie pri Medzinárodnom komitéte slavistov (Nové Vozokany 24. – 26. apríla 1989)*, Bratislava: Jazykovedný ústav Ľudovíta Štúra, 254-264.

Furdík, Juraj (2008), *Teória lexikálnej motivácie v slovnej zásobe* [Theory of lexical motivation in the lexis], Ološtiak, Martin (ed.), Košice: vydavateľstvo LG.

Galalaldeen, Ahmad and Hart, P. John (2007), 'Human Copper-Zinc Superoxide Dismutase and Familial Amyotrophic Lateral Sclerosis', in Uversky, Vladimir N. & L. Fink, Anthony (eds.), *Protein Misfolding, Aggregation, and Conformational Diseases, Part B: Molecular*

Conformational Diseases, New York: Springer Science + Business Media, LLC, 327-341.

Giannoni, Davide (2008), 'Medical writing at the periphery: The case of Italian journal editorials', *Journal of English for Academic Purposes* 7: 97-107.

Gilreath, Charles T. (1995), 'Resolving Term Disputes with Weighted Onometrics', in Wright, Sue Ellen & Strehlow, Allan (eds.), *Standardizing and Harmonizing Terminology: Theory and Practice, ASTM STP 1223*, Philadelphia: American Society for Testing and Materials, 25-52.

Gunnarsson, Britt-Louise (2009), *Professional Discourse*, London: Continuum.

Horecký, Ján (1956), *Základy slovenskej terminológie* [Essentials of Slovak terminology], Bratislava: Vydavateľstvo SAV.

—. (1967), 'O zásadách pri tvorení názvoslovia' [On the principles of formation of terminology], *Kultúra slova* 1/5: 129-132.

—. (1982), 'Systémový prístup k terminológii' [Systemic approach to terminology], *Kultúra slova* 16: 333-338.

International Statistical Classification of Diseases and Related Health Problems 10th Revision (2010) 'ICD-10', http://apps.who.int/classifications/icd10/browse/2010/en#/G12.2

ISO 1087-1. 2000 *Terminology work - Vocabulary Part1: Theory and Application*. Geneva: International Standards Organization.

ISO 5127. 2001 *Information and documentation - Vocabulary* Geneva: International Standards Organization.

Maher, John (1986), 'The development of English as an international language of medicine', *Applied Linguistics* 7: 206-218.

Masár, Ivan (1991), *Príručka slovenskej terminológie* [The Handbook of Slovak terminology], Bratislava: Veda.

Musil, Vladimír; Bozděchová, Ivana; Čech, Pavel; Lískovec, Tomáš; Stingl, Josef; Kachlík, David (2010), 'Anatomická terminologie - historie a aktuální problémy'. [Anatomical terminology – history and current problems], *ProInflow: Časopis pro informační vědy*, 2/1, Praha: Ústav informačních studií a knihovnictví filosofické fakulty UK, 58-75, available at http://pro.inflow.cz/anatomicke-nazvoslovi-historie-aktualni-problemy.

Poláčková, Gabriela (1992), 'Motivovanosť anglických, ruských a slovenských lekárskych termínov' [Motivatedness of English, Russian and Slovak medical terms], *Kultúra slova* 26/11-12: 338-346.

Štekauer, Pavol (to appear), 'Compounding from an onomasiological perspective', in ten Hacken, Pius (ed.), *The Semantics of Compounding*, Cambridge: Cambridge University Press.
Willis, Marjorie Canfield (2007), *Medical Terminology: A Programmed Learning Approach to the Language of Health Care*, Philadelphia: Lippincott Williams and Wilkins.
Wright, Sue Ellen (2006), 'Standards for the Language Industry', in ten Hacken, Pius (ed.), *Terminology, Computing, and Translation*, Tübingen: Gunter Narr Verlag, 19-40.

Dictionaries

OED (2014, 2015), *Oxford English Dictionary, Third edition*, John Simpson (ed.), www.oed.com.
Stedman (1997), *Stedman's Concise Medical Dictionary for the Health Professions*, John H. Dirckx (ed.), Baltimore: Williams & Wilkins.

CHAPTER FIVE

TRANSPARENCY OF NOMINAL COMPOUNDS IN MEDICAL ENGLISH: PROBLEMS IN THEIR TRANSLATION INTO SPANISH AND SLOVAK

NINA PATTON, MARÍA FERNÁNDEZ PARRA AND ROCÍO PÉREZ TATTAM

In English, compounding is a very productive word formation process, especially for N+N compounds. The interest of compounds for translators lies in that this level of productivity is not shared across languages, which means that N+N English compounds cannot always be translated by direct N+N equivalents into Spanish or into Slovak, for example. This poses a real problem, as not only will translators have to ensure they understand the compound fully before they translate it, but they will also need to select the most appropriate structure in the target language. In order to interpret the meaning of compounds fully, Jackendoff (2010: 417) insists that language users should focus on the semantic relations between compound constituents.

The aim of this paper is to ascertain whether there is a connection between semantic relations and the way they are translated into Spanish and Slovak. English, Spanish and Slovak represent three different language families, namely Germanic, Romance and Slavic, which means that there is potential for an interesting comparison of different word formation rules in all three languages. Compound productivity rates vary largely, resulting in variance of compound use in the languages, thus causing difficulties at the time of translating such structures. In particular, this paper will look at N+N compounds in medical English in dentistry, a subdiscipline of medicine which has been selected for its high content of specialized terminology and availability of sources.

We collected a representative sample of English N+N compounds from a reliable source and determined semantic relations for each of the entries as well as translations into Spanish and Slovak. We analysed the syntactic structures of the translations as we believed this would be a suitable, formal way of categorising them thanks to their reduced levels of ambiguity. We analysed the results with a special focus on frequency rates to determine whether there are patterns emerging. The analysis highlights the most frequent semantic relations in English compounds; the three most frequent ones are consequently looked at in further detail. We recorded the most frequent syntactic structures in Spanish and Slovak representing the most common translation choices and identified patterns. The emerging patterns confirm a connection between semantic relations and the choices translators made when faced with non-transparent N+N compounds in the source text.

We recommend further research to be undertaken to provide a detailed guidance applicable to translation practice. In any case, we have been able to produce an informed claim confirming a direct relation linking the semantic relations between compound constituents and the impact this has on the way compounds are translated into Spanish and Slovak. It also reaffirms how relevant the consideration of semantics is when interpreting compounds, especially for N+N compounds, which lack an explicit syntactic relation.

1 N+N compounds in the literature

The traditional literature from early to mid-20th century includes compounds in the study of morphology whilst highlighting their apparent syntactic properties (Bloomfield, 1933; Jespersen, 1942). There was very little analysis of the meaning until Lees (1960), adopting Chomsky's style of linguistics, analysed nominal compounds as derived from the so-called 'deep structure'. This approach required a sentence behind the meaning of each compound (e.g. *windmill* developed from 'a mill powered by the wind'). However, this became problematic when there was more than one eligible sentence, such as 'a mill that creates wind' for *windmill.* Half a century later, Jackendoff (2010: 428) resolves this by accepting multiple meanings, calling this phenomenon *promiscuity*, as shown in (1).

(1) a. ticket window 'a window at which tickets are bought'/ 'a window at which tickets are sold'
b. grammar school 'a school where grammar is taught'/ 'a school where grammar is learned or studied'

The above shows that it is rather the formulation of the relationships that is different, not the actual reality described by the interpretations. This concept stands in contrast with what Jackendoff calls *ambiguity* and is his understanding of the difficulty to interpret compounds, especially so-called *deictic* compounds (Venuti, 1995), which are spontaneously created by language users. For promiscuous non-lexicalized compounds, it is true that not only do they have multiple interpretations but these interpretations may also denote different realities, such as the examples in (2).

(2) a. boxcar 'car that carries boxes'
b. boxcar 'car that resembles a box'
c. boxcar 'car that serves as a box'

(3) a. pontoon bridge 'bridge supported by pontoons'
b. pontoon bridge 'bridge floating on pontoons'
c. pontoon bridge 'bridge made of pontoons'
d. pontoon bridge 'pontoons in a form of a bridge'

Promiscuous compounds which had been lexicalized can also offer various interpretations. In such cases, however, whichever interpretation is chosen by one particular speaker, will not affect the reality understood by another speaker, as for example in (3). Jackendoff argues that all of the above are acceptable because interpretations are embedded in meaning and that the meaning is a property of individual speakers. Preference for a specific meaning is "prejudice" (2010: 428). In conceptual semantics, the meaning of a compound is a function of the meanings of its constituents because semantics is an autonomous generative system, independent but not completely disconnected from syntax (2010: 425).

Jackendoff classes compounds as structures belonging to the so-called *protolanguage*, which is an initial stage of development of language that only involves its semantic and phonological aspects. In this environment, concepts are combined and thus compounds are built. An analogy is made with discourse, where syntax and morphology do not go beyond the boundaries of individual sentences and where additional 'connective tissue' is in existence though not necessarily explicit. This 'connective tissue' is the function of meanings of compound constituents. Jackendoff (2010: 436) lists fourteen classes of functions of meanings, explaining that some may be reversible or have several varieties bringing the overall number of individual relations to over 20. Examples include categories such as *kind of* which is reversible and thus materialises in two specific relations *N2 of kind N1* (e.g. *puppy dog, ferryboat*) and *N1 of kind N2* (e.g. *seal pup, bear cub*). The category *X serves as Y* involves the semantics of the constituent words and can be interpreted as *Y whose proper function is to function as an X*. Table 5-1 gives an impression of how many various relations this category can account for depending on what the proper function of the constituent is.

Category	***Example***	***Explanation***
N2 is a container	*photo album*	*album* contains *photographs*
N2 is a vehicle	*baby carriage*	*carriage* is a vehicle for *babies*
N2 is an article of clothing	*face mask*	*mask* is an article of clothing for *face*
N2 is itself a location	*movie theatre*	*theatre* is a location for *movies*
N2 is an incipient stage of something else	*grass seed*	*seed* is an incipient stage of *grass*
N2 is an agent or causer	*sanitation engineer*	*engineer* is an agent/causer for *sanitation*
N1 can describe the topic of the information	*success story*	*story* is about *success*

Table 5-1: Subcategories of *X serves as Y*

We considered Jackendoff's categories in principle and used his conceptualisation in the application of semantic relations. However, we avoided the use of the category *X serves as Y* in which the semantics of constituents play a crucial role. We did not wish to add an extra layer of analysis (e.g. N2 is a container, N2 is a vehicle, etc.), and thus we discarded the category *X serves as Y* for being largely generic and absorbing a high number of compounds, which would, naturally, result in a small number of categories. In order to allow a concise presentation of results and useful generalisations to be made, we adapted the list to resemble Plag et al.'s list (2008) with some additional semantic relations as they emerged during analysis. By doing this, those compounds which would be classed in *X serves as Y* were allocated a semantic relation category from Plag et al.'s list. This list had previously been used in an empirical study leading to conclusive results, which played an important role in our decision to opt for it instead of the theory-based list presented by Jackendoff. Both above-mentioned lists and how these relate to the final list we decided to adopt are outlined in the mapping in Appendix 1.

2 Methodology

The aim of this paper is to investigate whether a link can be established between semantic relations in medical English N+N compounds and their translations in Spanish and Slovak. The term *medical English* is widely used to refer to the language used in the field of medicine and by the professionals of health sciences and affiliated subject areas. However, it also includes the terminology used by patients, students, researchers, medical instrument manufacturers or even traders. The number of potential data sources and the variety of registers called for further specialization in order to achieve a cohesive and consistent data set which would be representative of a subfield within medical English. Dentistry, as a branch of medicine, was selected based on the basis of the availability of sources and specialist advice for translation.

Section 2.1 outlines the criteria based on which the English compounds were selected and the sources used. Section 2.2 provides a detailed description of the data set together with an overview of how the data set was analysed in terms of semantic relations between compound constituents. Finally, section 2.3 discusses the process of finding translations into Spanish and Slovak to achieve a set of trilingual entries and which additional information of analysis was recorded against the translations.

2.1 Compounds

We collected the compounds from Ireland (2010), which contains over 4,000 entries in total, representing key terms from a range of dental specialist areas, such as orthodontics or periodontology. The publication contained terminology from areas such as primary care, ethics and clinical research, which despite not being medical English terms are very closely related to dental sciences, as they are an inherent part of a day-to-day professional reality in dentistry.

Among the 4,000 entries, we focused on N+N compounds. These compounds in English were defined as compounds for which it was true that not only the overall category had to be a noun, but its constituents also had to be nouns, whether single words or compounds with the overall category of a noun. Such a rule excluded compounds like *aphtous ulcer* $[Adj+N]_N$ or *tieback* $[V+Adv]_N$ but included compounds such as *white spot lesion* $[[Adj+N]_N+N]_N$. No limit was set to the number of constituents.

Furthermore, we made a decision somewhat contrary to some traditional definitions of compounds (e.g. Bloomfield, 1933) to include compounds the constituent(s) of which are not strictly root forms, allowing for structures such as *health visitor* or *border moulding* to become part of the sample. We found that these structures represented over 10% of the data set, which indicates they are likely to be significant in medical English. In addition, compounds containing a proper noun, such as *Bimler appliance* and *Capdepont syndrome*, recorded over 16% of occurrences and were also included in the sample.

We found Spanish and Slovak translations for our final set of 492 English entries in bilingual dictionaries, parallel texts and with assistance of dentistry professionals. These sources are listed in Appendix 2. We then analysed the trilingual entries and categorized them in terms of discipline, number and distribution of constituents as well as additional information, such as synonyms, abbreviations and acronyms. These last three categories were not available for each entry but they were included in order to aid in translation. In the case of synonyms, if they met the criteria of nominal compounds as described above, such as *bite plane* and *bite plate,* both compounds were included as separate entries.

2.2 Semantic relations

Having compiled a list of compounds in the source language, the next stage required a categorization of the compounds in terms of semantic relations between the constituents. We adopted the list of semantic relations from Plag et al. (2008) within which Jackendoff's categories had been subsumed. Whilst it was necessary to work with a limited set of semantic relations to allow for the desired kind of analysis, the above-mentioned list was only a starting point and the project was open to introducing additional relations as they became relevant. Further classification was necessary for some categories (e.g. *N2 is located N1* was further divided into three subcategories), reverse direction was needed for some others (*N1 is like N2* and *N2 is like N1*) and one completely new relation was introduced - *N2 measures N1*. The final list of semantic relations with examples is shown in Table 5-2.

	Semantic relation	***Tokens***	***Frequency (%)***	***Example***
1	N2 causes N1	*4*	*0.62*	*air embolism*
2	N1 causes N2	*22*	*3.42*	*radiation caries*
3	N2 has N1	*19*	*2.95*	*cleft palate*
4	N1 has N2	*15*	*2.33*	*tooth mobility*
5	N2 makes N1	*3*	*0.47*	*sweat gland*
6	N1 makes N2	*1*	*0.16*	*Beeswax*
7	N1 made of N2	*1*	*0.16*	*baseplate wax*
8	N2 made of N1	*28*	*4.35*	*dentine bridge*
9	N2 uses N1	*54*	*8.40*	*colour therapy*
10	N1 uses N2	*3*	*0.47*	*biopsy needle*
11	N1 is N2	*5*	*0.78*	*amalgam waste*
12	N2 is N1	*15*	*2.33*	*buccinators muscle*
13	N1 like N2	*2*	*0.31*	*enamel rod*
14	N2 like N1	*42*	*6.53*	*ghost teeth*
15	N2 for N1	*150*	*23.33*	*amalgam carrier*
16	N1 for N2	*2*	*0.31*	*Framework*
17	N2 about N1	*15*	*2.33*	*germ theory*
18	N2 located in N1 – Human Intervention	*32*	*4.98*	*bone augmentation*
19	N2 located in N1 – Natural Process/Condition	*36*	*5.60*	*bone resorption*
20	N2 located in N1 – Object	*43*	*6.69*	*embrasure clasp*
21	N1 located in N2 – Natural Process/Condition	*4*	*0.62*	*stagnation area*
22	N1 located in N2 – Object	*4*	*0.62*	*basement membrane*
23	N2 during N1	*14*	*2.18*	*pregnancy epulis*
24	N1 during N2	*2*	*0.31*	*manipulation time*
25	N2 named after N1	*112*	*17.42*	*Bass technique*
26	N2 measures N1	*15*	*2.33*	*sugar clock*

Table 5-2: Semantic relations in nominal compounds

The two most common semantic relations are *N2 for N1* with 23.33% and *N2 is named after N1* with 17.42%. Very prominent is also the relation *N2 located N1,* which had been split in three more specific relations. However, if their frequency rates were to be added up, they would result in 17.26%.

Determining a semantic relation between compound constituents is subjective and compounds can be semantically ambiguous. Therefore, there were three raters involved in the allocation of semantic relations, each recording up to two possible semantic relations where necessary. Semantic relation 1 was the preferred option and semantic relation 2 was recorded as a possible option. Where there was an agreement by all three, the semantic relation was recorded automatically. Where two raters had recorded the same relation as their preferred option, which happened to be the third rater's possible option, this became the agreed relation in most cases. However, the third rater's preferred option was also given consideration and in 4% of cases, the third rater's choice was recorded. The chart in Figure 5-1 shows the proportion of agreement and ambiguous cases.

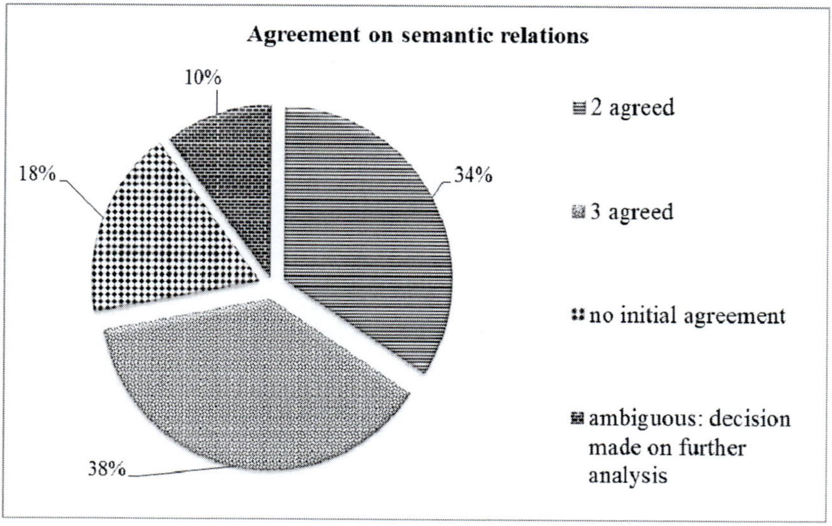

Fig. 5-1: Chart representing the three raters' agreement in assigning semantic relations

The ambiguous cases include cases where two raters recorded the same initial option, but after a discussion, the third rater's original choice was retained as well as cases where there was no initial agreement but after discussion, agreement was reached on a relation that had not originally been a preferred option of any of the raters. The relation that recorded the most agreement by three raters was *N2 named after N1*, followed by *N2 for N1* and *N2 uses N1*. As mentioned, there have been various compounds which all three raters found ambiguous, such as *group control* or *reference nutrient intake* and the relation most commonly recorded when there was either non-agreement or a difficulty in assigning a relation was *N2 for N1*, followed by *N2 is located in N1 – Human Intervention* and *N2 is located in N1 – Object*.

2.3 Translation triplets

The Spanish translations were sourced mainly from bilingual dictionaries and specialised websites. The main source for translations into Slovak was a team of professionals from the field of dentistry, namely a dental hygienist, dentist assistant and a dentist specializing in child dentistry. Amongst the team were both English and non-English speaking individuals who required various levels of assistance when clarifying the English terms. Original English definitions and illustrations, some of which were conveniently contained in the original source, were added and close communication with the team ensured there was no room for misinterpretation. In addition, we used online glossaries, encyclopaedia, professional clinics websites and other sources to find Slovak translations. Table 5-3 shows three examples of complete triplet data entries.

The next stage consisted of categorizing each Spanish and Slovak translation in terms of syntactic structure. For Spanish translations, the part of speech information of all constituents, including affixes, were noted. Where a noun was a proper noun, such as in *Trendelenburg position*, this was clearly noted. For prepositional phrases, the specific preposition was recorded, as we felt that the more detail is provided the more significant results can be discussed.

Similarly, for Slovak translations, the grammatical categories of all constituents were recorded, in addition to the grammatical case. There were several entries for which the same English word or compound was commonly used in Slovak and so this was also clearly identified. The decision to add the level of detail in both Spanish and Slovak was based on the realization that prepositions in Spanish and grammatical inflection in Slovak record a similar type of information, i.e. semantic relations in syntactic structures, so being specific would become crucial for this paper.

Term (en)	*abstinence syndrome*	*Albers-Schönberg disease*	*body mass index*
Definition (en)	Substance withdrawal	A congenital abnormality characterized by abnormally dense and brittle bones, which have a tendency to fracture. It may be associated with delayed tooth eruption, and osteomyelitis or necrosis following dental infection.	The weight of a person (in kilograms) divided by the square of the height of that person (in metres).
Discipline	Gen Med	Dent	Gen Med
Synonym		Osteopetrosis	
Acronym			BMI
Number of constituents	2	3	3
Syntactic structure (en)	N+N	N(proper)-N(proper)+N	N+N+N
Semantic relation (en)	N1 causes N2	N2 named after N1	N2 measures N1
Term (es)	*síndrome de abstinencia*	*enfermedad de Albers-Schönberg*	*índice de masa corporal*
Syntactic structure (es)	N+de+N	N+de+N(proper)-N(proper)	N+de+N+Adj
Term (sk)	*abstinenčný syndróm*	*Morbus Albers-Schönberg*	*index telesnej hmotnosti*
Syntactic structure (sk)	Adj+N	N(Lat)+N(proper)+N(proper)	N+Adj+N(Gen)

Table 5-3: Three examples of compounds with translations

3 Results

The main objective of this research was to identify if a relationship can be found between two variables: i) the semantic relation established between compound constituents in the source language and ii) the way compounds are translated. By 'the way compounds are translated' we were keen to identify any generalization which could be made and which could assist translators in their decision making when facing a nominal compound in English. We adopted a detailed description of the syntactic structure as a convenient means to identify the way compounds are translated in Spanish and Slovak.

In this section, we will discuss the way the most frequent categories of semantic relations have been translated and also whether the directionality of semantic relations matters in translation, i.e. whether it is relevant if the relation is *N1 for N2* or *N2 for N1*. Observing that it is indeed relevant for translation would imply that it is necessary to classify compounds not only in terms of the overarching semantic relation category (e.g. MADE OF) but also in terms of its direction (e.g. either *N1 made of N2* or *N2 made of N1*).

3.1 N2 for N1

Section 2.2 shows that the most common semantic relations are the following: *N2 for N1*, *N2 named after N1* and overarching *N2 is located N1* (see Table 5-2 for frequency rates). The high preponderance of *N2 for N1* can be explained in part by the multiple interpretations of the preposition *for*. It has, among others, the following applications: in favour of, with regard to, cause or purpose (Oxford English Dictionary). The pie chart in Figure 5-2 outlines the major groups of syntactic structures in Spanish we found to be used for this semantic relation. We have grouped these here for presentation purposes and the full break down of syntactic relations, including tokens, and examples in both languages (i.e. the original term in English and its translation equivalent in Spanish) can be found in Appendix 3. The group N in the pie chart represents both single or multiple noun structures (e.g. *separador* for 'tooth separator', and *banda matriz* for 'matrix band'). The category 'N+prep+N' contains combinations of nouns with any preposition other than *de* 'of' and *para* 'for' as these are treated as separate groups here.

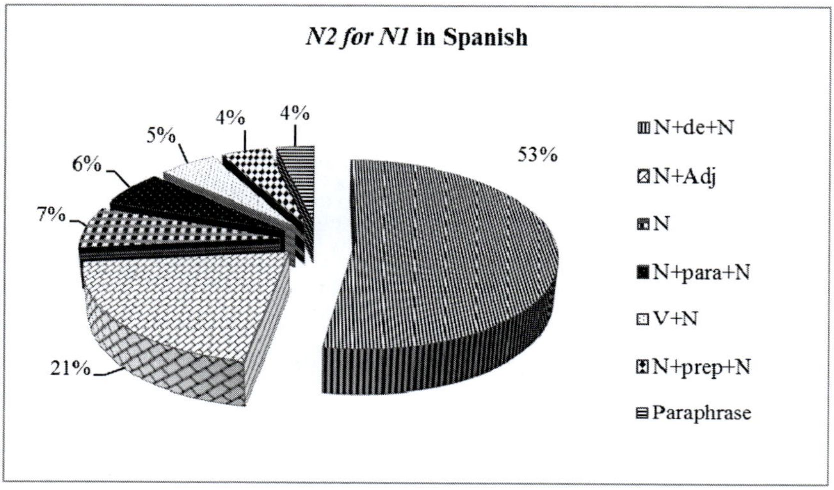

Fig. 5-2: Translations of the semantic category N2 for N1 in Spanish

It is easily identified that the most frequent way of translating *N2 for N1* English compounds is using an N+*de*+N (lit. N+'of'+N) structure in Spanish, which accounts for approximately 53% of the total translation equivalents. This shows that *de,* being a very widely used preposition, features in over half of the occurrences. This mirrors the wide range of applications of the preposition *for*. Having grouped all instances of translations with the Spanish preposition *para,* one of the usual translations of *for,* we found only seven occurrences (approximately 6%). For the other prepositions, such as *contra* ('against') or *en* ('in'), we did not record many tokens. We observed that in the few instances where minority prepositions were used in translation, they were used in limited ways. For example, the preposition *en* was not used to denote time but only location or manner, as can be seen in (4).

(4)	a.	fármaco en emergencia	lit. 'drug in emergency'
	b.	preparación cavitaria en túnel	lit.' cavity preparation in tunnel'

The second most frequent structure is N+Adj with over 20%. The adjectives are in almost all cases relational, as shown in (5) and very often are used to refer to a specific location, body part or area, as shown in (6).

(5) a. máscara facial lit. 'mask face$_{Rel_Adj}$'
b. balón dental lit. 'ball tooth$_{Rel_Adj}$'
c. auxiliar sanitaria lit. 'assistant healthcare$_{Rel_Adj}$'

(6) a. mouth mirror espejo bucal (lit. 'mirror mouth $_{Rel\_Adj}$')
b. tooth jewellery joya dental (lit. 'jewel tooth $_{Rel\_Adj}$')
c. pulp cap recubrimiento pulpar (lit. 'cover pulp$_{Rel_Adj}$')
d. cavity varnish barniz cavitario (lit. 'varnish cavity$_{Rel_Adj}$')
e. lip bumper aparato vestibular (lit. 'appliance passage$_{Rel_Adj}$')

The above would suggest that whilst the semantic relation of the English compound indicates purpose or function, expressed by the preposition *for*, this relation is not obvious in the translation, as relational adjectives in Spanish translation could have various connotations. For example *bucal* (lit. 'buccal', relating to the mouth) would generally be more likely to allude to something 'in the mouth' than 'for the mouth', *cavitario* (lit. 'cavitary', relating to the cavity) to 'in the cavity' rather than to 'for the cavity' and *vestibular* (lit. 'vestibular', relating to the vestibule) to 'in the lip area' rather than 'for the lip area'.

As for Slovak, the pie chart in Figure 5-3 shows a summary of our findings. Again, the variations of syntactic structures with smaller numbers of tokens have been grouped for presentation purposes and the full detail can be obtained from the table in Appendix 4. As can be observed, Adj+N is the most frequent structure found in translations of N+N compounds with over 40% of expressions, with the majority of adjectives being relational. The major category is followed by N+N (Gen), e.g. *odsávanie slín* (lit. 'suction of saliva', moisture control) with approximately 20%, followed by paraphrase, e.g. *os otáčania kĺbových kondylov mandibuly* (lit. 'axis of rotation of mandibular joint condyle', hinge axis) with 15%. The smallest category on the chart is the N+N (other than Gen) and represents a variety of N+N structures with components that are words in English, Latin, proper nouns or nouns in cases other than Genitive.

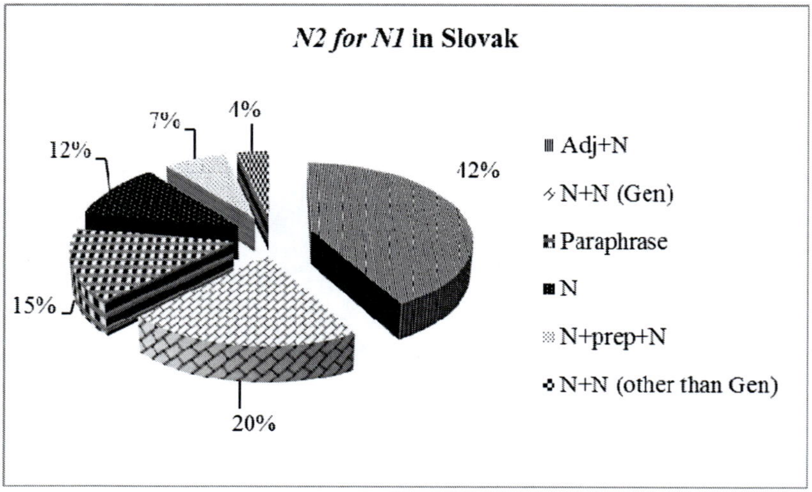

Fig. 5-3: Translations of the semantic category N2 for N1 in Slovak

In contrast with Spanish, where free translation of relational adjectives had the connotation of location, there is no evidence for a prevalence of any particular interpretation of relational adjectives in these structures, as shown in (7).

(7)	a.	mouthwash	ústna voda ('water in the mouth')
	b.	tooth separator	separačná gumička ('rubber which separates')
	c.	airway	dýchacie cesty ('way for breathing')
	d.	face shield	ochranný štít ('shield to protect')

The large variety of usage of relational adjectives in Slovak mirrors the number of applications of the preposition *for*. Thus an interesting observation presents itself, which is that a structure with the semantic relation *N2 for N1* containing a multi-purpose preposition is likely to be translated by equally multi-purpose structures, whether N+de+N when working with Spanish or N+Adj when translating into Slovak. This is a very high-level observation which would need further analysis, including a categorization of nouns in N+*de*+N instances in Spanish as illustrated in (8).

(8)	a.	expansion plate	prótesis de expansión N+de+$N_{Deverbal}$
	b.	air block	bloqueo de aire $N_{Deverbal}$+de+N
	c.	tooth paste	pasta de dientes N+de+N_{Pl}

Alternatively, for Slovak, the analysis would benefit from a classification of relational adjectives based on which structure they can be replaced by (e.g. *which*+V, *for*+V-*ing*, *to*+inf.) and from observing whether a pattern emerges linking any of these with a particular semantic relation category.

3.2 N2 named after N1

The second most frequent semantic relation of English medical compounds was *N2 named after N1*. In both Spanish and Slovak, there were clear indications that these structures are highly likely to be translated by structures containing the same proper noun. The reason is obvious, as the proper noun refers to the name of the brand, the scientist who discovered a disease or a patient who first exhibited symptoms indicative of a certain condition. They denote very specific entities and are often kept in translation.

In Spanish, this was the case for 88% of occurrences out of which the majority (over 78%) were N+*de*+N structures (N+*of*+N) or N+N expressions with nearly 17% of occurrences, as illustrated in (9a-b). Where no proper noun was used in the translation, a variety of N+*de*+N structures was predominant. A paraphrase is only used in two occurrences. An example is shown in (9c).

(9)	a.	Bass technique	técnica de Bass (lit. 'technique of Bass')
	b.	Bolam principle	prueba Bolam (lit. 'test Bolam')
	c.	Greene-Vermillion index	índice de la higiene bucal simplificado (lit. 'index of the hygiene oral simplified')

In Slovak, over 72% of *N2 named after N1* English compounds are translated using a variety of structures containing the same proper noun. With very few exceptions in which either i) there is a reference to a place rather than to a person in which a relational adjective as in (10a) would apply, or ii) the proper noun describes a technique, method or operation in which case a structure with the preposition *podľa* ('according to') would be used as in (10b), the proper nouns are in the possessive form, which coincides with genitive case as in (10c-e).

(10)	a.	Arkansas stone	arkansaský kameň (lit. 'Arkansas$_{Rel_Adj}$ stone')
	b.	Wildman flap	operácia podľa Wildmana (lit. 'operation according to Wildman')
	c.	Begg bracket	Beggov zámok (lit. 'Begg's lock')
	d.	Essig splint	Essigova spona (lit. 'Essig's splint')
	e.	Melkersson-Rosenthal syndrome	Melkersson-Rosenthalov syndrome (lit. 'Melkersson-Rosenthal's syndrome')

It is interesting to note that, in contrast to Spanish, in cases where the proper noun is not used, there is no other predominant structure to be used in translation. This is interesting as no direct solution can be suggested for translators; instead, it calls for more careful selection out of three structures which recorded similar frequency rates: paraphrases (7%), structures with a relational adjective (6%) and structures with nouns only (6%).

3.3 N2 is located in N1

The third most frequent semantic relation is *N2 is located in N1*. The decision to further categorize this relation into three subcategories was motivated mainly by the ambiguity of the generic one. Once the subcategories were made more specific, a significant increase in agreement amongst the raters was noted.

The results for the generic category reveal that two main structures in both languages are predominant, specifically N+Adj (45%) and N+*de*+N (44%) for Spanish and N+N_{Gen} (47%) and Adj+N (28%) for Slovak. The most frequent translations for the three subgroups of *N2 is located in N1* in Spanish and Slovak are illustrated in Figure 5-4 and Figure 5-5, respectively.

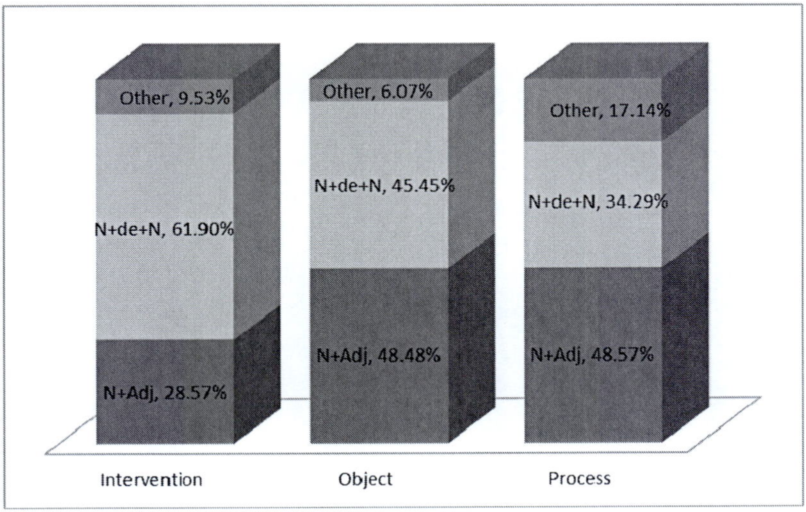

Fig. 5-4: Graphic representation of two most frequent syntactic relations in translation into Spanish of subcategories of N2 is located in N1 English compounds

It would appear that there is significantly more balance between the two most frequent options in Spanish than in Slovak. In Spanish, it is interesting to observe that the predominant syntactic structure is N+Adj in two subcategories: *Natural Process/Condition* and *Object.* However, there is a significant preponderance of N+*de*+N when the subcategory is *Human Intervention*, with 61.9% as opposed to 28.57% recorded for N+Adj occurrences.

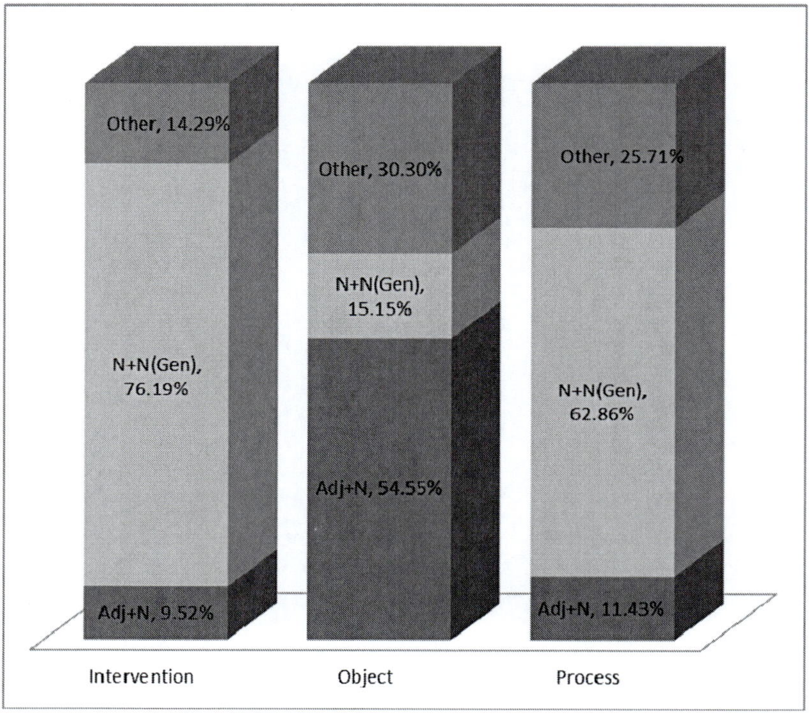

Fig. 5-5: Graphic representation of two most frequent syntactic relations in translation into Slovak of subcategories of N2 is located in N1 English compounds

The division into subcategories proves even more relevant in Slovak translation where there is one very clearly predominant category of syntactic structures for each subcategory. Similarly, two subcategories, though not the same as in Spanish, record a strong predominance of N+N(Gen) syntactic structures. It is the subcategory of *Object* which differs from the other two, noting a prevalence of Adj+N structures.[1]

[1] Here we do not take a strong position as to whether the N+N(Gen), (relational) Adj+N or prepositional structures are syntactic or morphological. From the perspective of translation practice, this distinction is not crucial.

3.4 Does directionality of semantic relations matter in translation?

It seems sensible to group semantic relations into families, so that generalizations can be made. However, it was of interest to determine whether there was a difference in terms of the prevalent syntactic structure used in translation when the semantic relations were analysed as families and when they were analysed as unidirectional relations (N1-N2 or N2-N1). The relations that do not have a reverse counterpart and have therefore been excluded from this part of the study are: *N2 about N1, N2 named after N1, N2 is located in N1 – Human Intervention* and *N2 measures N1*. In addition, the relation families marked by MADE OF and MAKES, which only recorded one token in one of the directions, have been excluded due to the lack of sufficient data for comparison.

In the majority of cases, two main syntactic relations have been identified for translation into each language. The most interesting cases were when there was a discrepancy between the structure most prevalently used across the relation family (using combined data of e.g. *N1 for N2* and *N2 for N1*) and a unidirectional relation from that same family (e.g. *N2 for N1*). Besides the imbalance of frequency rates amongst the two main syntactic structures, the appearance of a third structure or a lack of a second structure implying a monopoly of a single syntactic relation were also of interest.

As illustrated in Figure 5-6, the family CAUSE shows a discrepancy in Spanish as it would appear that N+*de*+N is the most prevalent syntactic structure when combined data is considered. However, this is not the case in *N2 causes N1* where N+Adj seems prevalent.

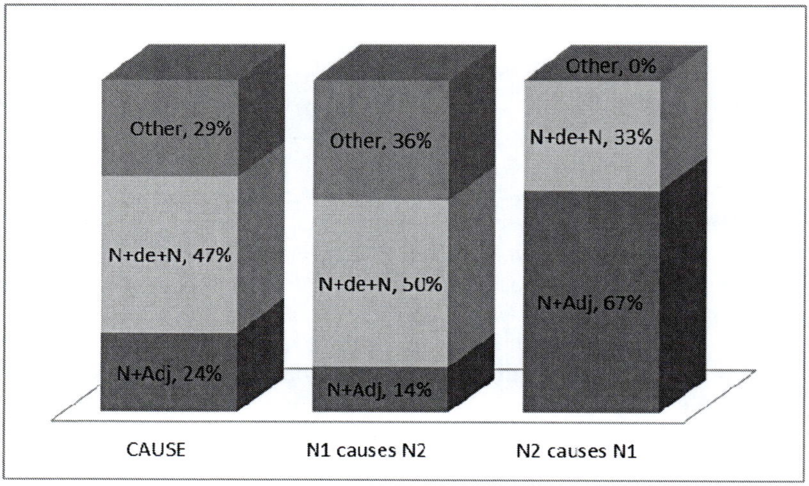

Fig. 5-6: CAUSE in Spanish

For DURING, Slovak translations show an equal number of tokens between the syntactic realizations for *N1 during N2* which contrasts with the prevalence of Adj+N when data are considered collectively for the family, as shown in Figure 5-7.

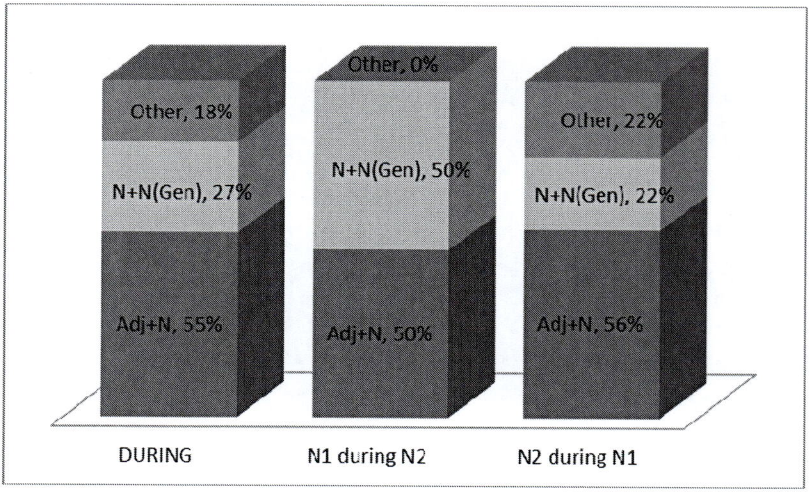

Fig. 5-7: DURING in Slovak

Another interesting observation is that a third syntactic structure appears to be prevalent when a relation is considered unidirectionally but loses this status in the combined data. An example of this is the family FOR in Slovak, where the structure N comprises 50% of tokens in *N1 for N2*, but does not feature as one of the two predominant structures when the entire family FOR is considered, as shown in Figure 5-8. This loss of prevalence status is due to an imbalance of tokens between *N1 for N2* and *N2 for N1*. It is therefore important that these are considered one by one, each direction separately.

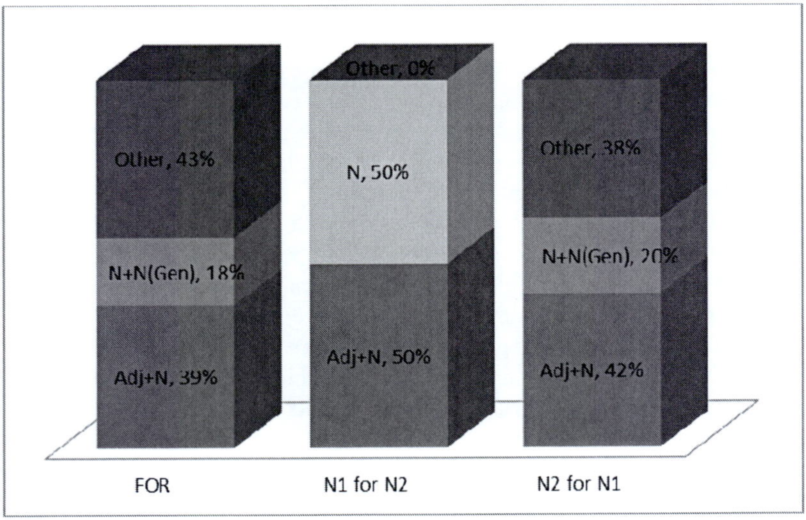

Fig. 5-8: FOR in Slovak

In addition, it would appear that if the number of tokens is relatively balanced between the two unidirectional semantic relations, such as in *N1 has N2* and *N2 has N1*, with 11 and 16 tokens respectively, the ratio of tokens of structures in translation is also relatively balanced in both languages. The fact that there are two structures with similar frequency rates makes it harder for the translators as it does not highlight one mainstream syntactic structure. It would therefore be advisable for translators to take special care when facing similar cases to ensure the correct structure is adopted.

The family LOCATED IN is one of the largest in terms of number of occurrences within our data set and has been compiled out of three subcategories as mentioned in detail in section 3.3. The division into three subsets was justified by the varying results across the three subsets. One could thus expect that a similar pattern of varying results would be obtained from the directionality test. As the focus here was on the direction, the tokens from the three subsets (*Human Intervention, Natural Process/Condition* and *Object*) were added up and grouped by direction only. Surprisingly, the Spanish translations recorded nearly a 50:50 ratio for the two mainstream syntactic structures used, which would imply that for this semantic relation family, the direction is not relevant in translation.

4 Conclusion

The varying productivity of N+N compounds in the three languages (English, Spanish and Slovak) results in the need for alternative structures when translating N+N English compounds. The objective of this paper was to establish whether a relationship can be found between two variables: i) the semantic relation between N+N compound constituents and ii) the way the compounds are translated into Spanish and Slovak. Having followed Jackendoff's framework for interpreting compounds (2010) and Plag et al.'s (2008) list of semantic relations, we focused on semantic relations between compound constituents.

Once N+N English compounds from dentistry were collected, they were analysed by three raters in terms of their semantic relations. The analysis showed that the structures which are likely to be used in majority as a translation of English nominal compounds were N+*de*+N and N+Adj in Spanish, and N+N(Genitive) and Adj+N in Slovak. Similarly, there are a few categories of semantic relations that are predominant and in our data set these were *N2 for N1*, *N2 named after N1* and *N2 is located N1*.

It was of interest here to determine if N+N compounds from medical English (as opposed to general English) presented any specifics, whether in terms of the interpretation of source compounds or their translation. Some specific properties were observed already at the stage of allocation of semantic relations. For example, the category NAMED AFTER was observed to be a prominent relation. Spanish and Slovak translations maintained the proper noun most of the time. Section 3.2 explains why this is not to be taken as a rule. In addition, it was noted that some compounds had been translated using Latin or English words for denominating syndromes, instruments or procedures. For example, *collapse therapy* translates as *pneumonotorax* into Slovak and *veneer crown* translates into Spanish as *corona veneer.* The semantic relation here does not seem to play a role but it is important to note that the use of neo-classical formations and original English words is something a translator may encounter in translating medical English. They should be aware that leaving a constituent in its original English form (*lip bumper* translated as *lip bumper* in Slovak) or using a Classical form (*pedicle flap surgery* translated as *gingivoplastia* in Spanish) is acceptable due to the widespread use of English, Latin and Greek in scientific disciplines, medical science not being an exception.

The results seem to suggest that there is a link between the semantic relation of the English compound and the syntactic structure of the translation. It is true that the two mainstream syntactic structures described above predominated. However, there is no absolute predominance of either of them and the fact that different semantic relations correlate with different syntactic structures supports the existence of such a link.

We have included the presentation of results for the three main categories. A similar type of information has been found for all semantic relations listed in Table 5-1. However, the fact that almost 60% of compounds have been considered in the analysis of the three major categories vindicates our decision to focus on these, as they account for a large proportion of problems a translator could encounter when translating medical texts.

Further research might be carried out on the relation *N2 for N1* allowing for a subdivision of the compounds based on the various applications of the proposition *for*. This would be in accordance with the 'proper function of' as explained by Jackendoff and it is believed that this would be likely to reveal results that could serve as a guidance to professional translators.

The extent to which the syntactic structure of translations truly and accurately represents the notion of 'the way the compounds are translated' would also benefit from further investigation. One could argue that knowing what words are used in translation is more important than knowing the syntactic structure. Sometimes brand new lexical items come into play, meaning that some of the source compound constituents are not used in translation at all. For example *reservoir bag* translates in Spanish as *bolsa de respiración* ('breathing bag') where the constituent *reservoir* does not appear in the translation. Similarly, the translation into Slovak *kyslíkový rezervoár* ('oxygen reservoir') drops the constituent *bag*. An analysis that would combine the syntactic structure and the indication of source constituents 'recycling' might yield interesting results.

References

Bloomfield, Leonard (1933), *Language*, New York: Holt.

Ireland, Robert (2010), *Oxford Dictionary of Dentistry*, Oxford: Oxford University Press.

Jackendoff, Ray (2010), *Meaning and the Lexicon: The Parallel Architecture 1975-2010*, Oxford: Oxford University Press.

Jespersen, Otto (1942), *A Modern English Grammar on Historical Principles: Part VI Morphology*, Copenhagen: Munksgaard.

Lees, Robert B. (1960), *The Grammar of English Nominalizations*, Bloomington: Indiana University.

Plag, Ingo; Kunter, Gero; Lappe, Sabine & Braun, Maria (2008), 'The role of semantics, argument structure, and lexicalization in compound stress assignment in English', *Language* 84: 760-794.

Venuti, Lawrence (1995), *The Translator's Invisibility: A History of Translation,* London: Routledge.

Appendix 1

Mapping of semantic categories: Jackendoff (2010), Plag et al. (2008) and the list used in this paper

	Semantic relation Jackendoff*		**Semantic relation (Plag et al)**		**Semantic relation (Patton et al)**
		1	N2 causes N1	1	N2 causes N1
1	N2 that is caused by N1	2	N1 causes N2	2	N1 causes N2
2	X has Y	3	N2 has N1	3	N2 has N1
		4	N1 has N2	4	N1 has N2
3	X makes Y	5	N2 makes N1	5	N2 makes N1
		6	N1 makes N2	6	N1 makes N2
				7	N1 made of N2
4	X is composed of Y	7	N2 made of N1	8	N2 made of N1
5	X is made out of Y				
		8	N2 uses N1	9	N2 uses N1
		9	N1 uses N2	10	N1 uses N2
6	Y is (also) an X	10	N1 is N2	11	N1 is N2
				12	N2 is N1
7	N2 similar to N1	11	N1 like N2	13	N1 like N2
				14	N2 like N1
		12	N2 for N1	15	N2 for N1
				16	N1 for N2
		13	N2 about N1	17	N2 about N1

	Semantic relation Jackendoff*		Semantic relation (Plag et al)		Semantic relation (Patton et al)
8	X at/in/on Y	14	N2 is located at/in…N1	18	N2 located in N1 - Human Intervention
				19	N2 located in N1 - Natural Process/Condition
				20	N2 located in N1 - Object
		15	N1 is located at/in…N2	21	N1 located in N2 - Natural Process/Condition
				22	N1 located in N2 - Object
		16	N2 during N1	23	N2 during N1
				24	N1 during N2
		17	N2 named after N1	25	N2 named after N1
				26	N2 measures N1
9	N1 classifies N2				
10	N2 of/by N1				
11	X is a part of Y				
12	X kind of Y				
13	X serves as Y				
14	X protects Y from Z				

*Jackendoff's semantic relations are expressed as functions. Where variables X and Y are used to describe the function above, the function is reversible.

Appendix 2

Syntactic structures of Spanish translations for *N2 for N1* English compounds

Ref.	Syntactic structure (es)	Translation (es)	Term (en)	Tokens	Frequency rate (%)
1	N	separador	tooth separator	5	4.46
2	N(affix)+N	gingivoplastia	pedicle flap surgery	1	0.89
3	N+Adj	barniz cavitario	cavity varnish	22	20.53
4	N+Adj+*en*+N	preparación cavitaria en túnel	tunnel preparation	1	0.89
5	N+Adj+*para*+N	retractor elástico para mejillas	cheek retractor	1	0.89
6	N+*anti*+N	vacuna anti-caries	caries vaccine	1	0.89
7	N+*contra*+N	protección contra las radiaciones	radiation protection	1	0.89
8	N+*de*+N	medio de contraste	contrast medium	49	43.75
9	N+*de*+N(pl)	cepillo de dientes	toothbrush	3	2.68
10	N+*de*+ N(proper)	fórmula de Black	instrument formula	1	0.89
11	N+*de*+N+Adj	gancho de acción reversa	back-action clasp	4	3.57
12	N+*de*+N+*de*+N	tarjeta de control del tratamiento	treatment card	1	0.89

Ref.	Syntactic structure (es)	Translation (es)	Term (en)	Tokens	Frequency rate (%)
13	N+N+*de*+N	cera registro de mordida	bite registra-tion wax	1	0.89
14	N+*en*+N	fármaco en emergencia	emergency drug	2	1.79
15	N+N	banda matriz	matrix band	2	1.79
16	N+*para*+N	apoyo para el dedo	finger rest	3	2.68
17	N+*para*+N(pl)	fresa para fisuras	fissure bur	3	2.68
18	Paraphrase	jeringa para la inyección de materiales de impresión	impression material syringe	4	3.57
19	V+N	portapelícula	film holder	3	2.68
20	V+N(pl)	abrebocas	mouth pop	3	2.68

Appendix 3

Syntactic structures of Slovak translations for *N2 for N1* English compounds

Ref.	Syntactic structure (sk)	Translation (sk)	Term (en)	Tokens	Frequency rate (%)
1	Adj+Adj+N	snímateľný orto-dontický aparát	tooth positioner	3	2.68
2	Adj+N	ústna voda	mouth-wash	44	39.29
3	Adj+N+N(Gen)	priame prekrytie drene	pulp cap	1	0.89
4	Adj+N+*na* +N(Acc)	ochranná maska na tvár	face mask	2	1.79
5	N	matrica	matrix band	7	6.25
6	N(Affix)+N	gingivo-plastika	pedicle flap	2	1.79
7	N(Agent)+N(Gen)	roztvárač úst	cheek retractor	2	1.79
8	N(EN)	bond	cavity varnish	2	1.79
9	N(EN)+N(EN)	lip bumper	lip bumper	1	0.89
10	N(EN-brand)	optragate	lip retractor	2	1.79
11	N(Lat)+N(Lat)	logopédia	speech therapy	1	0.89
12	N(Proper)+N	rochettova dlaha	abutment splint	1	0.89

Ref.	Syntactic structure (sk)	Translation (sk)	Term (en)	Tokens	Frequency rate (%)
13	N+Adj(Gen)+ Adj(Gen)+ N(Gen)	odľahčenie hornej totálnej náhrady	relief area	1	0.89
14	N+Adj(Gen)+ N(Gen)	prevencia zubného kazu	caries prevention	4	3.57
15	N+*medzi*+N(Instr)	medzery medzi zubami	Spillway	1	0.89
16	N+N(Gen pl)	odsávanie slín	moisture control	5	4.46
17	N+N(Gen)	napínač matrice	matrix retainer	8	7.14
18	N+N(Gen) +N(Gen)	vizualizácia sanácie chrupu	preview model	2	1.79
19	N+N(Instr)	liečba náhradou	replace-ment therapy	1	0.89
20	N+*na*+N	chránič na zuby	mouth guard	3	2.68
21	N+*na*+N+N(Gen)	pilník na korene zubov	bone file	1	0.89
22	N+*proti*+Adj(Dat) +N(Dat)	vakcína proti zubnému kazu	caries vaccine	1	0.89
23	Paraphrase	os otáčania kĺbových kondylov mandibuly	hinge axis	17	15.18

Appendix 4

Translation sources

Adamicová, Katarína (2008), *Biopsia kože*, Martin: Mgr. Libuša Chrásteková – Vydavateľstvo.

Celec, Peter (2012), *Ako publikovať v medicínskych vedách,* Bratislava: Univerzita Komenského Bratislava.

Collins Spanish-English English-Spanish Dictionary (2009), 9th ed., Glasgow and New York: Collins.

Drgoňa, Ľuboš (2008), 'Liečba infekcií vyvolaných vírusom herpes zoster u imunokompromitovaných pacientov', *Ambulantná terapia* 6: 228-229.

Ďurkovský, Juraj & Bolješíková, Elena (2008), *Rádioterapia zhubných nádorov*, Bratislava: Liga proti rakovine SR.

Gurčík, Ladislav (2010), 'Neskorá neuroborelióza či postboreliový syndróm?', *Nerologická prax* 11:402-405.

Hanobik, František; Krajči, Jozef; Gurský, Ján; Proněková, Martina; Micheľ, Radoslav; Korbová, Zuzana & Malinková, Gabriela (2012), *Zborník z medzinárodnej vedeckej konferencie Quo vadis hospic,* Bratislava: VŠZaSP sv. Alžbety.

Kaplan, Steven M. (2008), *Diccionario Jurídico Inglés-español, Español-inglés*, Alphen aan den Rijn: Kluwer Law International.

Kelz, Rochelle K. (1997), *Delmar's English-Spanish Pocket Dictionary for Health Professionals*, Albany: Delmar Publishers.

Koviačik, Jozef & Beniač, Martin (2005), *Pružnosť a pevnosť pre špeciálne inžinierstvo*, Žilina: Žilinská Univerzita.

Krahulec, Boris (2005), 'Obezita a niektoré faktory prostredia podporujúce vznik metabolického syndrómu', *Cardiology* 14: 161-165.

Minčeffová, Marianna (2011), *Informovanosť verejnosti o možnosti paliatívnej starostlivosti*, Brno: Masarykova Univerzita.

Olšovská, Katarína; Živčák, Marek; Hunková, Elena & Dreveňáková, Petra (2013), 'Hodnotenie fotosyntetických charakteristík a rezistencie na vysokú teplotu pri tetraploidných genotypoch pšenice (Triticum L.)', *Journal of Central European Agriculture* 14: 767-780.

Prevendárová, Jitka (2004), *Rodinná terapia a poradenstvo*, Bratislava: OZ Sociálna práca.

Rovenský, Jozef; Buchvald, Dušan & Rádiková, Žofia (2012), 'Koža a reumatické ochorenia', *Dermatologická prax* 6: 112-122.

Ruiz Albrecht, Erich & Ruiz Albrecht, Francisco (2000), *F.Ruiz Torres Diccionario de términos médicos*, Valladolid: Zirtabe.

Scasso, Mauro; Morra, Stefano & Costa Luca (2007), 'Prístup certifikácie EWF podľa EN ISO 3834: Nástroj manažmentu na zvládnutie európskych smerníc o zváraných výrobkoch', *Zváranie* 56: 18-24.

Šepitka, Peter (2007), *Ranné teórie svetla Newton – Huygens*, Žilina: Žilinská Univerzita.

Springhouse English and Spanish Medical Words and Phrases (1999), 2nd ed., Springhouse (PA): Springhouse Corporation.

Sršeň, Štefan; Sršňová, Klára & Zibolen, Mirko (1998), 'Vrodené vývinové chyby kardiovaskulárneho systému z hľadiska genetických faktorov a dysmorfogenézy', *Bratislavské lekárske listy* 12: 652-658.

Stedman Diccionario bilingüe (1999), Maryland, Argentina, Madrid: Editorial médica panamericana.

Štefanková, Ivana & Fabián, Juraj (2005), 'Diagnostika porúch prekrvenia a dysfunkcie myokardu', *Via practica* 2: 183-188.

Talapková, Renáta; Hudeček, Jan; Šinák, Igor; Kubisz, Peter; Hlinka, Ľuboš; Patkaňová, Lenka; Zeleňák, Kamil & Laca, Ľudovít (2010), 'Autológna transplantácia kmeňových buniek pre záchranu ischemickej končatiny – predbežné výsledky', *Vaskulárna medicína* 2: 89-92.

Váleková, Ľubica (2005), 'Poruchy zrážania krvi', *Via practica* 2: 311-315.

Zamorano Pino, Ximena & Valenzuela Aránguiz, Vladimir (2011), 'Caso Clínico: Prótesis Fija Plural a Corona Tres Cuartos. Solución Antigua a Problema Actual', *Revista Dental de Chile* 102: 32-34.

Žiaková, Eva (2014), *Ako nájsť zmysel života v sociálnej práci s rizikovými skupinami*, Košice: Univerzita Pavla Jozefa Šafárika.

Dental professionals

Helena Olenočinová – Dentist Assistant, Dental Practice Jonek Dent

Iveta Samcová – Dental Hygienist, Dental Practice Jonek Dent

Dr. Daniela Némethová – Dentist, Dental Practice MUDR. Daniela Némethová

Online sources

Acta Odontológica Venezolana (no date), http://www.actaodontologica.com/ (viewed 12 Oct. 2014).

A-Z encyklopédia – slovenská online encyklopédia (no date), http://www.az-encyklopedia.info/ (viewed 26 Oct. 2014).

CAO-Blog 3eraño Odontología (2014), http://3erodontourg.wordpress.com/ (viewed 19 Oct. 2014).

CardioSalud – Comisión Honoraria para la Salud Cardiovascular (no date), http://cardiosalud.org/ (viewed 4 Sept. 2014).
Clínica dental Dr. Juan Balboa (2014), http://www.juanbalboa.com, (viewed 19 Oct. 2014).
Clínica Donnay (no date), http://www.clinicadonnay.com (viewed 19 Oct. 2014).
Clínica Odontológica López y Calviño (no date), http://www.clinicalopezycalvino.com/ (viewed 19 Oct. 2014).
Čo je Bachova terapia? (2010), http://www.bachova-terapia.sk/ (viewed 10 Sept. 2014).
Dental A2Z, Quality Dental Supplies Affordable Prices – EN ISO 13485:2012 Certified Company (2014), http://dentala2z.co.uk/P es%2019/10/2014D9191/ (viewed 19 Oct. 2014).
Depósito dental Den-thel (no date), http://www.dent-thel.com/ (viewed 19 Oct. 2014).
Diccionario de cáncer – National Cancer Institute (2012), http://www.cancer.gov/diccionario (viewed 19 Oct. 2014).
Diccionario Médico (no date), http://diccionario.medciclopedia.com/ (viewed 4 Sept. 2014).
Diccionarios.com (2011), http://www.diccionarios.com/detalle.php?palabra=splint&dicc_98=on (viewed 4 Sept. 2014).
Drogový informačný portal (2012), http://www.infodrogy.sk/ (viewed 11 Sept. 2014).
Epicentro- un sitio de apoyo al aprendizaje de la epidemiología (no date), http://escuela.med.puc.cl/recursos/recepidem/index.htm (viewed 19 Oct. 2014).
Facultad de Estudios Superiores Iztacala, UNAM, México (2012), http://www.iztacala.unam.mx (viewed 19 Oct. 2014).
Facultad de Odontología, Universidad Nacional de Colombia (no date), http://www.odontologia.unal.edu.co/ (viewed 19 Oct. 2014).
Forestadent – German precision in Orthodontics (2015), http://www.forestadent.com/forestadent-us/ (viewed 19 Oct. 2014).
Glosario de terminus en protésis total removable (2014), http://www.sdpt.net/completa/dicionario.htm (viewed 19 Oct. 2014).
IQB: Mediclopedia (2013), http://www.iqb.es/diccio (viewed 19 Oct. 2014).
Laboratorio Ortodoncia – Dental – Ortoplus (2014), http://www.ortoplus.es (viewed 19 Oct. 2014).

Lekári Zdravie Lekárstvo Online Zdravotníctvo (2015), http://www.lekarionline.sk/ortopedia/diskusia/acp-liecba-krvnou-plazmou (viewed 26 Sept. 2014).
Medigraphic – Indice de Revistas Médicas Latinoamericanas (no date), http://www.medigraphic.com/ (viewed 19 Oct. 2014).
MedlinePlus – Información de Salud de la Bilbioteca Nacional de Medicina (2015), http://www.nlm.nih.gov/medlineplus/spanish/ (viewed 4 Sept. 2014).
Odontologos.com.co – la comunidad de salud oral ás grande de Colombia (no date), http://www.odontologos.com.co/ (viewed 4 Sept. 2014).
Orphanet (2015), http://www.orpha.net/consor/cgi-bin/index.php (viewed 10 Sept. 2014).
Ortodoncia Málaga – Dr Manuel Román (2011), http://www.ortodonciamalaga.com/ (viewed 19 Oct. 2014).
Pre Alergikov (no date), http://www.prealergikov.sk/ (viewed 4 Oct. 2014).
Pregunta al dentist online (2013), https://www.propdental.es/dentista/ (viewed 4 Sept. 2014).
Revista Latinoamericana de Ortodoncia y Odontopediatría (no date), http://www.ortodoncia.ws/ (viewed 4 Sept. 2014).
Revistas Médicas Cubanas (no date), http://bvs.sld.cu/revistas/ (viewed 19 Oct. 2014).
Slovak Resuscitation Council (2014), http://www.srr.sk/ (viewed 2 Oct. 2014).
Slovak society of cardiology (2008), http://www.cardiology.sk/ (viewed 2 Oct. 2014).
Spa dental (2015), http://spadental.do/ (viewed 4 Sept. 2014).
Statistical office of the Slovak republic (2014), http://slovak.statistics.sk (viewed 14 Sept. 2014).
Suvison - The reference source for the world dental community (2015), http://www.suvison.com/ (viewed 19 Oct. 2014).
Tratamientos dentales: información, precios, beneficios y riesgos (no date), http://tratamientodental.es/ (viewed 4 Sept. 2014).
Univerzitná knižnica Prešovskej Univerzity (2015), http://www.pulib.sk/web/kniznica/strana/nazov/uvodna-strana (viewed 14 Oct. 2014).
Vicerrectorado de Política Científica e Investigación (2015), http://investigacion.ugr.es/pages/etica (viewed 16 Oct. 2014).
Výskumný Ústav zváračský (2012), http://www.vuz.sk/ (viewed 14 Sept. 2014).

Zdravie.sk – 500,000 ľudí mesačne sa spolieha na naše informácie (2015), http://www.zdravie.sk/ (viewed from 10 Sept. to 14 Oct. 2014).

CHAPTER SIX

WORD FORMATION STRATEGIES IN TRANSLATED POPULAR MEDICAL TEXTS IN TURKEY

SEVDA PEKCOŞKUN

Popular medical texts are written to inform the general public about health issues, trending topics and new approaches in medicine. Therefore, these texts are expected to be understandable and applicable for lay people in order to be beneficial in daily life. As full comprehension of a passage is closely related to the understanding of the terms in the text, analysing word formation strategies of terms in popular medical texts contributes to answering the question of to what extent popular medical texts truly address their target readers. In this chapter, I have used a parallel corpus that covers translated popular medical texts published within a certain period in Turkey and I have determined the frequencies of applied word formation strategies in the texts. The texts under the category of health on the BBC website (www.bbc.co.uk) and their Turkish translations on the BBC Turkish website (www.bbc.co.uk/turkce) have been analysed as per medical/health terms. The statistics reveal which word formation strategies in translated texts within the corpus were chosen more often and the data also shed light on the understanding of the translation strategies adopted. Analysing the word formation strategies used in translated texts also contributes to determining their success in reaching the target readership.

1 Popular Medical Texts

Medical texts could be classified as per their style, content, terminology and linguistic choices taken by the author of the relevant text. Newmark (1988:153) suggests three levels of language for medical texts based on medical terms used in the texts:

- **Academic texts:** These texts are marked by Latin and Greek words associated with academic papers. *agranulocytosis*, *hyperlipidaemia*, *nephrotoxicity* are some examples used in academic medical texts.
- **Professional texts:** Formal terms which are generally used by experts are included in the texts. *Occlusion*, *perivascular*, *pustular* are examples of professional terminology.
- **Popular texts:** They include terminology understood by laymen and the terms also have some alternatives. *Mumps*, *school sores* and *whooping cough* are terms encountered in popular texts.

As understood by the definitions and examples above, academic and professional medical texts have their own jargons and they are understood by a limited number of people comprised of academicians, professionals, specialists, medical experts and staff. On the other hand, popular texts include terms generally understood by individuals in the society from different social, economic, cultural and educational backgrounds.

Professional medical texts carry distinctive features at word and sentence levels which are not familiar to the general public. However, target readers of popular texts are comprised of a huge readership from different social levels. It is expected that medical information should be accessible, understandable and applicable for laymen in order to be applied in daily life. Popular medical texts are able to contribute to the solution of this challenge. These texts are published in health magazines, newspapers, brochures and websites to inform the public about health issues.

Popular medical texts are generally written with simpler terminology and structures in order to be adequately understood by target readers. While professional medical texts include special terminology and professional knowledge, popular texts include basic information and explications. The scope of this chapter is limited to popular medical texts and their translations.

2 Translation of Popular Medical Texts

Reiss (2000:26) categorizes texts as content-focused (informative), form-focused (expressive) and appeal-focused (operative) as per the language dimension. According to this classification, informative texts, such as lectures and course books, focus on giving information on facts and transferring the content; aesthetic effect and author's style become prominent in expressive texts such as poems and plays; and operative texts, such as advertisements, are written to take response from the readership. Medical texts (academic, professional or popular) which have the purpose of informing people (layman, expert, medical student, etc.) about a specific medical issue generally carry the features of informative texts.

Popular medical texts could be classified under the genre of popular scientific texts. Grasping the attention of the reader is an important objective of popular scientific texts. The writer attaches great importance to arousing the curiosity of the reader; semantic and stylistic characteristics which could be perceived as obstacles by readers are not welcome.

According to the model introduced by Löning (1981), there are four main levels of communication. These are professional to professional (e.g. scientific texts), professional to semi-professional (e.g. course books), professional to non-professional (e.g. patient education books) and non-professional to non-professional (e.g. popular science texts) (cf. Herget & Alegre, 2009).

Another classification on the basis of levels of communication is proposed by Pearson (1998:35-38). She classifies communicative settings as expert to expert (e.g. legal documents), expert to initiates (e.g. subject-specific textbooks), relative expert to uninitiated (e.g. popular science journals) and teacher-pupil (e.g. instruction manuals) communication. These communicative settings put forward by Pearson correspond to professional to professional, professional to semi-professional, non-professional to non-professional and professional to non-professional communication levels respectively when compared to Löning's classification.

According to these classifications, popular medical texts fall into the categories of professional to non-professional and non-professional to non-professional communication (or teacher-pupil communication and relative expert to uninitiated). For instance, patient education publications are written by medical experts to inform the public about a health issue. This could be an example of professional to non-professional communication. A simpler language and popular terms are preferred in those texts in order to be understood by target readers. Non-professional to non-professional texts are encountered in magazines, health bulletins and newspapers. They include terms understandable by people from different backgrounds. Source and target texts used in the study fall under the scope of non-professional to non-professional communication. As the objective of this communication is to convey the message to the target reader in a transparent and comprehensible way, term formation strategies adapted by the translator play an important role in the understandability of the target text.

As with source texts, it is expected from the target texts to address the readers by using transparent expressions that will not cause confusion. That serves as the aim of the translation of these texts.

According to Skopos Theory, put forward by Vermeer (2000:221-232), a translatum (the resulting translated text) is a consequence of the skopos (aim or purpose of a translation) and the translator, as an expert, is responsible for the final translation while taking the skopos into consideration. Thus, the translator is a key player in the process of communication between cultures and the production of the target text. Reiss and Vermeer (1984:113) state that target text should be coherent for target readers, given their circumstances and knowledge (cf. Munday, 2008: 80).

As underlined in Skopos Theory, which shifts its focus from the source to the target, the translator has instructions prior to translating and one text could be translated in many different ways to suit many different purposes (cf. Pym, 2010:49).

As we all know, translation is more than a linguistic transfer between two languages. Besides linguistic transfer, the nature of the translation involves communication, because while a source text functions in the source culture and source literary system; the target text functions as an independent text in connection with other texts within the target corpus. The task of the translator gains importance at this point. S/he shall strive to choose the most appropriate strategies in order to produce a functional and acceptable target text at an optimal level while taking the purpose (skopos) of the target text into consideration. This process requires the knowledge of the translator about the target readership in order to take necessary decisions as per the skopos of the translation. As Ammann (2008:59) states, the question "what the objective of the text is" is closely related to another question "For whom the translation is made".

As mentioned before, popular medical texts are informative texts written to inform the general public about health issues. Because of the fact that they address different social groups, and lots of people from different educational and cultural backgrounds have quick access to these texts, different groups of target text readers want the translator to meet their expectations by producing a target text in accordance with the standards of the target readership. For instance, a translator may not choose a medical term which is only understandable among medical doctors in a popular medical translation. Even if there is a high medical expression in the source text, the translator shall make the necessary adaptations and transfer the expression into target language in a communicative, functional and acceptable way. Therefore, the translation reaches its purpose which is to inform people about medicine/health issues. The translator plays a crucial role in creating a translatum that can be perceived as a fluent text by target readers as if written in their own language.

The skopos of the translation determines the translation methods that are to be used by the translator in order to produce a functionally adequate result. Two questions are crucial for the translator; why a source text is to be translated and what the function of target text will be? (cf. Munday, 2008:79).

As understandability of the terms in popular medical texts contributes to the fluency, coherence and clarity of the text, term formation strategies in the translations of popular medical texts are to be determined in accordance with the skopos.

3 A Review of Translation Procedures

Translators use different methods within the process of translating in order to make the target text explicit. The translator formulates the target text by adopting the methods which s/he has chosen. Vinay & Darbelnet (1995:30) describe the starting point of the translator as reading the message and then they claim that translators consider the impression of the target they want to reach. They explain two general translation strategies as **direct translation** and **oblique translation**. While direct translation methods are identified as **borrowing**, **calque** and **literal translation**; oblique translation methods include **transposition**, **modulation**, **equivalence** and **adaptation**. (cf. Vinay & Darbelnet, 1995:30-42). Generally speaking, the methods of borrowing and calque are mostly applied to units closer to a lexical basis, while other methods are used at both lexical and textual levels. Direct translation strategies make the translation more source-oriented and oblique translation strategies make the target text more target-oriented.

Vinay & Darbelnet (1995:41) present a table involving these seven strategies and exemplify the procedures on the levels of lexis, structures, and the message. In other words, the procedures may be applied to words, compounds and the semantic content.

I will briefly explain the translation procedures put forward by Vinay & in some examples chosen from the parallel corpus in sections 3.1 to 3.7.

3.1 Borrowing

According to Vinay & Darbelnet's model (1995:31), borrowing is the simplest of all translation methods. The translator applies this method in order to overcome a lacuna (gap in the target language). The word of the source language is directly transferred into the target language in borrowing.

Newmark (1988:81-82) uses the term *transference* for transferring a word in source language (SL) into the target language (TL). While he uses *transference* as direct transfer of SL units, he suggests the term *naturalisation* as a translation procedure. Naturalisation involves transference; but the translator adapts the SL word first to the normal pronunciation and to the normal morphology of the TL. Some examples from the parallel corpus are given in (1).

(1)	a.	musculoskeletal (EN)	muskuloskeletal (TR)
	b.	pelvic (EN)	pelvik (TR)
	c.	cerebellum (EN)	serebellum (TR)
	d.	cortex (EN)	korteks (TR)
	e.	cardiovascular (EN)	kardiyovasküler (TR)
	f.	obesity (EN)	obezite (TR)
	g.	autism (EN)	otizm (TR)

The words seen in (1) are terms translated into Turkish via the procedure of borrowing. According to Newmark's classification, the terms are naturalised, that is to say, they are adapted to Turkish pronunciation and morphology. For instance, one of the Turkish vowels *ü* which is not present in English alphabet is used in the translation of *cardiovascular (*TR *kardiyovasküler)* and the letter *x* in the word *cortex* is transferred into *ks* in the target word *korteks*, because of the fact that the letter *x* is not present in the Turkish alphabet. However, there are expressions transferred into Turkish via pure borrowing such as *sperm* (EN 'sperm'), *fibula* (EN 'fibula'), *bilateral* (EN 'bilateral'), *neonatal* (EN 'neonatal') and *vitamin* (EN 'vitamin').

Vinay & Darbelnet (1995:32) point out that some well-established, generally older borrowings that are widely used are no longer seen as borrowings and they have become the components of target language nomenclature. This assessment is also valid for Turkish as the target language with regard to medical terms. For instance, *kanser* (EN 'cancer'), *prostat* (EN 'prostate'), *stres* (EN 'stress'), *virüs* (EN 'virus'), *astım* (EN 'asthma') and *gastrit* (EN 'gastritis') are some of the borrowed words which are widely used and understood by Turkish people from different backgrounds.

The procedure of borrowing cannot always result in a transparent and understandable target text even if the source terms are naturalised. In other words, all borrowed expressions do not make sense to target readers unless they have sufficient knowledge about the relevant medical issue. Therefore, the translator should take the skopos of the translation into consideration and think twice on using borrowed terms. For instance, *musculoskeletal pain* and *pelvic pain* are transferred to the TL as *muskuloskeletal ağrı* and *pelvik ağrı*. *Ağrı* is the literal translation of the source word *pain*. It could be easily understood by Turkish readers. However, borrowed expressions as *muskuloskeletal* and *pelvik* are not familiar expressions to target readership from different parts of the society. Although the terms are naturally used and understood among medical staff, readers of popular medical texts may not comprehend the meaning of those borrowed terms. That is to say, unless the borrowed expression is widely known by target readers, the translator should prefer the appropriate derivation in the target lexicon generally known by the public while translating popular texts. As mentioned before, adapting a target-oriented approach accords with the skopos of popular medical texts. The translator also had better be aware of the differences between source and target cultures when making decisions. Therefore, it is appropriate to ask: "Is the procedure of borrowing an appropriate one used in the translations of popular medical texts from English to Turkish?"

As discussed in Section 4 below, borrowing is a popular and widely-used translation procedure chosen by the translators of popular medical texts within the corpus. Therefore, the appropriateness of the borrowing procedure between SL and TL should be discussed.

Toury (1995:54) states that translation is subject to constraints of several types on various levels in its socio-cultural dimension. Translation is an activity affected and also motivated by restraints created by the target society.

> Translation is a kind of activity which inevitably involves at least two languages and two cultural traditions, i.e., at least two sets of norm-systems on each level. Thus, the "value" behind it may be described as consisting of two major elements:
>
> (1) being a text in a certain language, and hence occupying a position, or filling in a slot, in the appropriate culture, or in a certain section thereof;

> (2) constituting a representation in that language/culture of another, pre-existing text in some other language, belonging to some other culture and occupying a definite position within it [Toury (1995:56)].

Therefore, the target text in the target culture does not have a secondary position as per its source text in the source culture. Toury (1995:56-57) defines translation as a norm-governed activity and the norms influence the choices of the translator. While adherence to source norms results in an adequate translation, adherence to target norms determines the acceptability of the target text.

Due to the fact that translated popular medical texts easily accessed by the general public in magazines, websites, newspapers, brochures, etc. have some objectives such as informing the individuals from different sections of the society and giving some advice on health issues, the translation should be transparent and acceptable as much as possible. That is to say, a target-oriented text is perceived as more coherent and reasonable by target readers. As understanding the message in popular medical texts is highly dependent on the comprehension of the terms that are used, choosing the appropriate equivalents of terms in the target language gains great importance. Given that the translation is realized between such languages as English and Turkish which have various differences on lexical, linguistic and cultural levels, the translator's preferences for procedures to guarantee the acceptability of the target text become crucial. I try to explain this assumption below.

According to Radu (2008:145) "98% of medical terms have Latin and Greek origins and have their own rules of word building with distinctive characteristics" in medical English. Dirckx (2006: APP 9) expresses a similar idea:

> Until the early modern era, the language of medicine consisted largely of Latin terms, many of them containing stems derived or adapted from Greek. Today Latin remains the official language of anatomic terminology and taxonomic nomenclature.

As understood from the quotations above, Latin and Greek terms still greatly influence English medical terminology.

When we turn attention to English as used for general purposes, we see that Latin and Greek influences are still present. Wikipedia (2014) mentions a computerized survey of about 80,000 words in the *Shorter Oxford Dictionary* (3rd edition) by Thomas Finkenstaedt and Dieter Wolff (1973) where it is estimated that 28.24% of English words are of Latin origin and 5.32% of the words are of Greek origin.

Therefore, it is possible to say that English readers are familiar with medical terminology influenced by Greco-Latin elements. For instance, the adjective *anaerobic* encountered in the corpus is presumably known by an English readership; that is to say, the term is familiar to the source culture. Therefore, an English reader does not have any difficulty in comprehending the term and the compounds including the term such as *anaerobic infection.* If the reader does not understand the term, s/he may look up the word in a general English dictionary. For instance, *anaerobic* is defined as "(of an organism or process) requiring the absence of or not dependent on the presence of oxygen" in the *Collins Dictionary* (2014).

When the term is translated into Turkish as *anaerobik* via the method of borrowing, most Turkish readers get confused about the meaning of the word because of its incompatibility with the features of Turkish as the target language. The term does not appear in general Turkish dictionaries. It only appears in the *Turkish Dictionary of Science and Art* published by the Turkish Language Association. That is to say, a word that is widely understood by the source culture is only understandable to medical specialists in the target culture. Therefore, it could be said that when the borrowed term does not make any sense to the target reader, it is the translator's task to choose the appropriate procedure in order to render the word in a more functional way. For instance, the translator could use an approved literal equivalent of the term, or prefer an accepted equivalent in the TL with the borrowed term, as illustrated in (2).

(2) a. Yet fears among health workers are high and have risen further after the recent death from the virus of the head of the haematology division, Ayman Hamdan Simi, at Jeddah's King Fahd Hospital.[1]

b. Bu korkular, Cidde'deki Kral Fahd Hastanesi **hematoloji (kanbilim)** bölümü başkanı Ayman Hamdan Simi'nin geçtiğimiz günlerdeki ölümü sonrasında arttı.[2]

c. *lit.* 'These fears, in Jeddah King Fahd Hospital after the **haematology (blood science)** division head Ayman Hamdan Simi's death in recent days, increased.'

As seen from the source and target texts in (2), the translator uses a borrowed term *hematoloji* (EN 'haematology'), but adds a literal equivalent chosen from the Turkish lexicon which could be truly

[1] Source text; http://www.bbc.com/news/world-middle-east-27337627

[2] Target text;
http://www.bbc.co.uk/turkce/haberler/2014/05/140512_suudiarabistan_salgin

understood by target readers as *kanbilim* (kan: EN 'blood', bilim: EN 'science'). Therefore, the translator is the decision maker on using borrowed terms while taking the attitudes of target society into consideration.

3.2 Calque

Vinay & Darbelnet (1995:32) define the procedure *calque* as a special kind of borrowing. The TL borrows an expression form of the SL, but then translates its elements literally. That is to say, the structure or expression in SL is transferred into TL via literal translation. Calques are classified into two groups: The translator preserves the syntactic structure of the TL, but introduces a new mode of expression in lexical calque. However, a new construction into the TL is introduced in structural calque (1995:32).

(3)	a.	surfer's eye (EN)	sörfçü gözü (TR)
	b.	super-clotting (EN)	süper-pıhtılaşma (TR)

In (3a), the procedure of lexical calque is used. A new mode of expression which could be perceived as odd is used in Turkish translation. A Google search for *sörfçü gözü* gives 6 results, all of them in translated texts. On the other hand, the medical equivalent of *surfer's eye*; *pterygium* (TR *pterigium*) is mostly used in original Turkish texts. Furthermore, pterygium which could be accepted as a professional term is generally known as *bird's wing* (TR *kuş kanadı*) among the general public in Turkey. Therefore, *sörfçü gözü* is a novel and unfamiliar expression for Turkish speaking readers.

In (3b), a procedure of structural calque is used. It introduces a new construction into Turkish. Use of hyphenated expressions such as *süper-pıhtılaşma* (EN 'super-clotting') is not so common in Turkish. Compounds in Turkish generally do not include a hyphen.

Newmark (1988:84) names the procedure of calque as "through-translation". According to his definition, through-translation refers to the literal translation of common collocations, names of organizations, the components of compounds and the phrases. He also suggests that through-translations should only be used when they are already recognized terms in TL.

3.3 Literal Translation

Literal translation is word-for-word translation. It means the direct transfer of an SL element into grammatically and idiomatically appropriate TL expression (cf. Vinay & Darbelnet, 1995:33). In (4) are some examples of literally translated expressions into Turkish from the corpus.

(4)	a.	infectious diseases (EN)	bulaşıcı hastalıklar (TR) *bulaşıcı* (EN 'infectious') *hastalık-lar* (EN 'disease-s')
	b.	white blood cells (EN)	akyuvarlar (TR) *ak* (EN 'white') *yuvar-lar* (EN 'blood_cell-s')
	c.	symptom (EN)	belirti (TR)
	d.	external hemorrhaging (EN)	dış kanama (TR) *dış* (EN 'external') *kanama* (EN 'hemorrhaging')

Literal translation could be applied as a method to the extent that target expressions are truly understood by readers. While analysing term formation procedures in translated texts, I have incorporated the procedure of calque into the literal translation procedure in the study, because both of them constitute word-for-word translation; that is to say, calque is also a literal translation method. Another reason for this choice is that sometimes it becomes difficult to trace calques in Turkish, because some expressions have closely incorporated into the TL and it is hard to determine whether an expression is a pure calque or literal translation.

3.4 Transposition

Transposition means the replacement of one word class with another without a change in the meaning of the message (cf. Vinay & Darbelnet, 1995:36). Newmark (1988:85) defines *shift* (Catford's term) or *transposition* (Vinay & and Darbelnet's term) as a translation procedure that involves a change in the grammar from SL to TL. In (5) are the terms translated with this procedure.

(5)	a.	patients with anorexia (EN)	anoreksik hastalar (TR) *anoreksik* (EN 'anorexic') *hasta-lar* (EN 'patient-s')

b. people with autism (EN) | otistik insanlar (TR)
otistik (EN 'autistic')
insan-lar (EN 'people')

The translator prefers adjectives such as *anoreksik* (EN 'anorexic') and *otistik* (EN 'autistic') in the TL for the nouns *anorexia* (TR 'anoreksiya') and *autism* (TR 'otizm') in the SL. This is a transposition according to Vinay & Darbelnet's classification. It is most probable that the translator prefers this change between parts of speech in order to support the fluency of the target text.

3.5 Modulation

Vinay & Darbelnet (1995:36) define modulation as a variation in the form of the message by a change in the point of view. When an SL expression is translated literally or even via transposition, it could be still considered unsuitable or awkward in the TL. Then, the translator applies modulation.

(6) a. cortisol (EN) | böbreküstü bezlerinin salgıladığı hormon (TR)
böbreküstü bez-lerinin (EN 'of adrenal gland-s')
salgıladığı (EN 'excreted')
hormon (EN 'hormone')

b. donor matching (EN) | doku uyumu (TR)
doku (EN 'tissue')
uyumu (EN 'compatibility')

As seen in (6a) *cortisol* is transferred into TL as *böbreküstü bezlerinin salgıladığı hormon* (EN 'hormone excreted by adrenal glands'). This is a part-whole modulation in Vinay & Darbelnet's terms, because cortisol is one of the hormones excreted by adrenal glands and there are other hormones such as aldosterone and adrenalin. *Donor matching* is translated into TL as *doku uyumu* (EN 'tissue compatibility'). *Donor* means a person who voluntarily gives her/his blood, tissue, organ etc. for use in the treatment of another person, so tissue could be accepted as a part of the donor. (6b) also involves part-whole modulation. The translator prefers modulation when literal translation could be perceived as unacceptable by target readers even though the translation is grammatically correct. That is to say, the translator uses a more common expression used in Turkish while changing the point of view.

3.6 Equivalence

Equivalence means describing the same situation in SL by using different stylistic and structural methods in TL. Therefore, equivalent texts are produced (Vinay & Darbelnet, 1995:38). (7) is an example from the parallel corpus.

(7) night terrors (EN) karabasan (TR)

The literal translation of "night terrors" is *gece korkuları*, but it does not make much sense to target readers; so *karabasan* (EN 'black sinking') is chosen which is a cultural and an idiomatic expression in Turkish. However, the message of the source expression does not change in TL. *Karabasan* means nightmares or fearful dreams in Turkish. Therefore, in (7) we have a Turkish expression whose etymology is entirely independent of the English expression it is a translation of.

3.7 Adaptation

Vinay& Darbelnet (1995:39) consider the procedure of adaptation as the extreme limit of translation. If the type of situation in the SL is not known in the target culture, the translator applies the procedure of adaptation and creates a new situation in the TL which s/he considers as being equivalent.

The translation of one text within the corpus that is used deserves attention. The title of the source text published on June 29th, 2014 is "Organ Transplants: 'Supercooling' keeps organs fresh". The text is about an innovation that aims to extend the life of organs (BBC News, 2014). The project is conducted by some researchers and one of these researchers is a Turkish doctor, Korkut Uygun. His name and statements appear in the source text. The target text titled "Derin Soğutma Nakil Öncesi Organ Ömrünü Uzatabilir" and published on June 30th, 2014 includes some adaptations (BBC Türkçe, 2014).

It is seen in the target text that there is an emphasis on the Turkish researcher. For instance, a statement by Korkut Uygun appears at the beginning of the target text, while the statements made by the researcher appear in the middle of the source text. Another adaptation is made in the sub-heading of the text. There is a sub-heading as "Supercool" in the source text. This heading is changed into "Ekipte Türk doktor var" (EN 'There is a Turkish doctor in the group') in the target text. The nationality of the researcher is not mentioned in the source text, but it is clear that the translator emphasizes this point in order to arouse the curiosity of target readers by making a target-oriented translation. This is not a cultural adaptation and the translator does not produce a new situation in the TL. S/he makes an adaptation at the textual level by adding an emphasis on the Turkish researcher without changing the content and message of the source text. Another adaptation chosen from the corpus is (8).

(8) a. Inspired by traditional cuisine of countries such as Greece, Spain and Italy, the Mediterranean diet has long been associated with good health and fit hearts.[3]
b. Yunanistan, İtalya, **Türkiye** ve İspanya gibi ülkelerin mutfaklarıyla özdeşleşen Akdeniz mutfağının kalp sağlığı için faydalı olduğu uzun süredir dile getiriliyor.[4]
c. *lit.* 'Greece, Italy, **Turkey** and Spain like countries' cuisines identified with Mediterranean cuisine for heart health to be beneficial for a long time is being voiced.'

As seen in (8), the translator makes an addition to the target text. The word *Türkiye* (EN 'Turkey') is added to other Mediterranean countries Greece, Spain and Italy. This decision does not change the main paradigm of the text, but could be accepted as an adaptation.

4 Corpus Study: Statistics on Translation Procedures

I have compiled and used a parallel corpus including 100 source texts and 100 target texts in the study. Medical terms encountered in the texts have been classified into two groups: one-word terms and multi-word terms. I analysed 634 terms (257 one-word; 377 multi-word) retrieved from the corpus and classified them as per translation methods. Figure 6-1 represents the translation procedures used, resulting in one-word terms in Turkish within the corpus.

[3] Source text; http://www.bbc.com/news/health-27470115
[4] Target text;
http://www.bbc.co.uk/turkce/haberler/2014/05/140520_akdeniz_diyeti

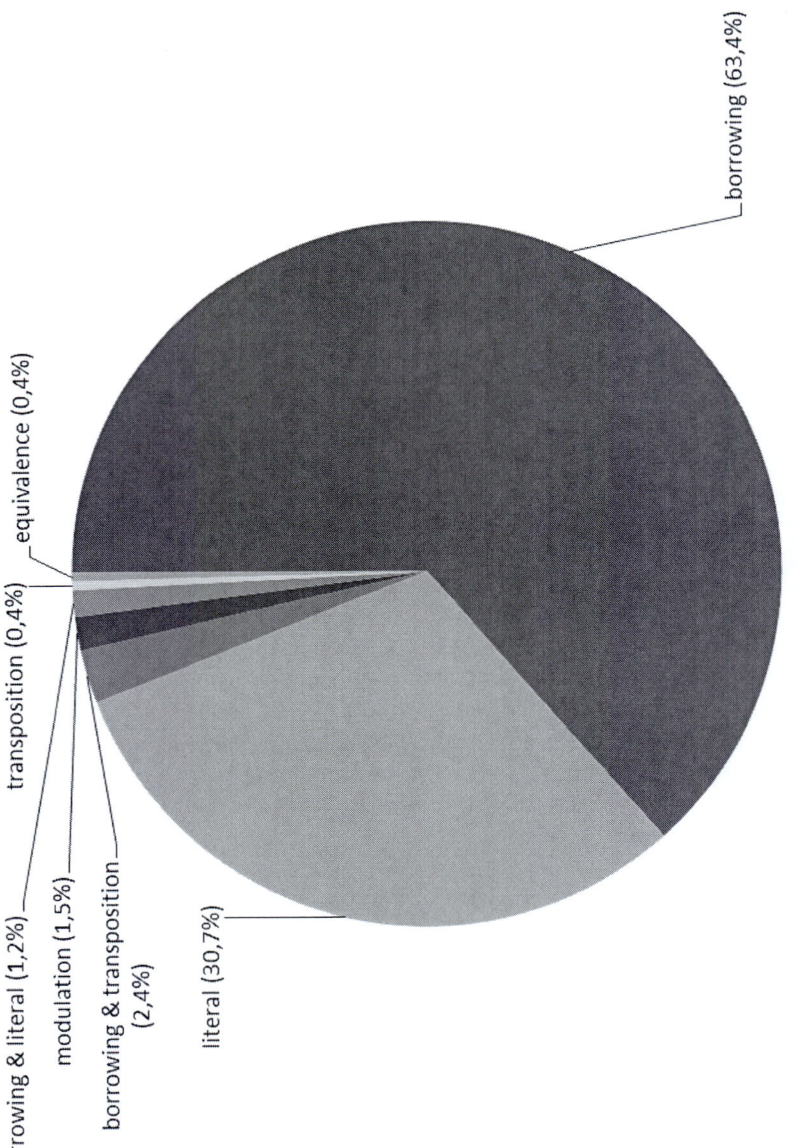

Fig. 6-1. Translation procedures of one-word terms

As seen from the graph, borrowing is the most widely used procedure (63.4%). Most borrowings are compatible with Turkish grammatical and morphological rules (what Newmark calls *naturalisation*). Borrowing is followed by literal translation (30.7%). Other methods (modulation, transposition and equivalence) are rarely used. Adaptation which is not a commonly used procedure in popular scientific texts such as popular medical texts is not observed at word level. There are also some hybrid strategies such as borrowing-literal and borrowing-transposition procedures, as in (9).

(9) a. biosecurity (EN) biyokoruma (TR)
biyo (EN 'bio'; borrowing)
koruma (EN 'security'; literal)
b. nanosphere (EN) nanoküre (TR)
nano (EN 'nano'; borrowing)
küre (EN 'sphere'; literal)

Figure 6-2 shows procedures used for multi-word terms encountered in the Turkish part of the corpus. Translation procedures used for multi-word terms differ from the ones for one-word terms. A combination of literal and borrowing (39%) is the most widely chosen procedure by translators. As seen from Figure 6-2, 33.2% of the multi-word terms are translated just literally. The third widely-used procedure is borrowing (14.9%). Modulation, transposition, borrowing-modulation combination, literal-modulation combination, transposition-modulation combination, literal-transposition combination, and borrowing-transposition combination procedures are the least preferred procedures. Some examples for hybrid procedures for multi-word terms are shown in (10).

(10) a. computerized tomography (EN)
bilgisayarlı tomografi (TR)
bilgisayarlı (EN 'computerised'; literal)
tomografi (EN 'tomography'; borrowing)

b. regenerative medicine (EN)
rejeneratif tıp (TR)
rejeneratif (EN 'regenerative'; borrowing)
tıp (EN 'medicine'; literal)

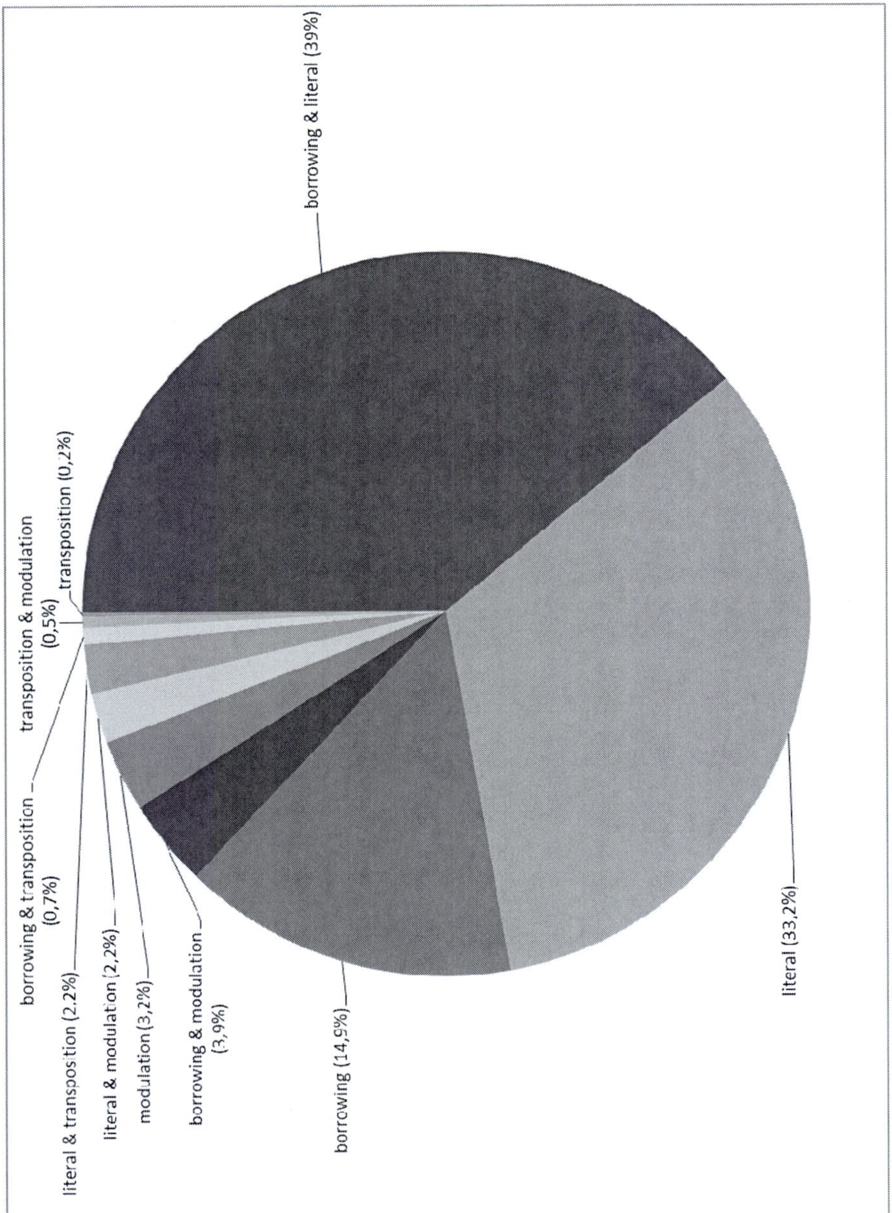

Fig. 6-2. Translation procedures of multi-word terms

c. psychotic event (EN)
psikotik rahatsızlık (TR)
psikotik (EN 'psychotic'; borrowing)
rahatsızlık (EN 'event'; modulation)

d. musculoskeletal pain (EN)
muskuloskeletal ağrı (TR)
*muskuloskelatal (*EN 'musculoskeletal'; borrowing)
ağrı (EN 'pain'; literal)

5 Case Study: A Questionnaire about the Medical Understanding of the General Public

An online mini-questionnaire was conducted in Turkish (target language) in order to determine which procedures used in the process of translating medical terms are more understandable and transparent for readers from different backgrounds. People were asked to answer some questions about the public understanding of popular medical terms. 183 people answered the questions. The participants came from different age groups and education levels and they were all Turkish native speakers.

It is observed that 58.5% of the respondents are partly interested in popular medical/health texts and 64.5% of respondents find popular medical texts that they encounter in daily life partly clear. The respondents were asked some questions in order to observe the influence of lexical choices on the understanding of popular medical/health texts. The results may reveal which translation procedures contribute more to the intelligibility of the popular medical texts.

In each question, I asked the respondents: "According to you, which sentence/sentences is/are (more) understandable?" There were two alternative sentences in each question. The respondents were free to opt for just one alternative or both. Also, they were able to express that they could not understand either of the alternatives.

All the questions were asked in the same manner; but the intention behind asking the questions was different. In the first question, my intent was to see how borrowing and literal translation of the terms affect the understanding of popular medical texts. The two alternative sentences given for this question were (11a-b).

(11) a. Kognitif bozukluklar, kardiyovasküler hastalıklar, diyabet ve demans gibi rahatsızlıkların düzenli egzersizle giderilebileceği yönünde kanıtlar var.

b. Zihinsel işlev bozuklukları, kalp damar hastalıkları, şeker hastalığı ve bunama gibi rahatsızlıkların düzenli egzersizle giderilebileceği yönünde kanıtlar var.
c. EN 'There is some proof that illnesses such as cognitive disorders, cardiovascular diseases, diabetes and dementia could be relieved with regular exercise.'

83.2% of respondents found sentence (11b) clearer. (11b) includes literal equivalents of English terms such as *bilişsel* (EN 'cognitive'), *kalp damar* (EN 'cardiovascular'), *şeker hastalığı* (EN 'diabetes'), and *bunama* (EN 'dementia'). However, (11a) includes the same terms translated with borrowings such as *kognitif* (EN 'cognitive'), *kardiyovasküler* (EN 'cardiovascular'), *diyabet* (EN 'diabetes'), *demans* (EN 'dementia'). Regarding the result given above, the translator had better reconsider using borrowed terms in order not to produce a hardly comprehensible target text while translating popular medical texts.

In the second question, I examined the transparency level of older, widely-accepted borrowings and their literal equivalents. The two alternative sentences given for the question were (12a-b).

(12) a. Lösemi hastalarında apandisit görülmesi sık karşılaşılan bir durum değildir; ancak her iki durumun da gözlemlendiği vakalar ölümcül olabilir.
b. Kan kanseri olan kişilerde kör bağırsak iltihabı görülmesi sık karşılaşılan bir durum değildir; ancak her iki durumun da gözlemlendiği vakalar ölümcül olabilir.
c. EN 'It is common that people with leukemia do not suffer from appendicitis simultaneously; however having both diseases at the same time could be fatal.'

Sentence (12a) includes borrowed terms which are widely known and used in the target language, such as *lösemi* (EN 'leukemia') and *apandisit* (EN 'appendicitis'). Sentence (12b) contains literal equivalents of the English terms in the target language, such as *kan kanseri* (EN 'leukemia') and *kör bağırsak iltihabı* (EN 'appendicitis'). 41.5% of respondents found both sentences clear. However, 30.1% preferred (12b) and 24.1% (12a). Taking into account that a wide majority of respondents found both alternative sentences clear, it could be inferred that the transparency levels of older, widely-accepted borrowings and their literal equivalents in target language are similar. Therefore, the translator who is aware of the target readers' attitudes, approaches and words that are in daily use in the society knows the borrowed terms which are widely accepted by the society and can use them in addition to literal equivalents.

In the third question, I examined to what extent a brief explanation of a borrowed term affects the intelligibility of the text.

(13) a. Yapılan konferansta palyatif tıp yöntemlerinin yaygınlık kazanmasının gerekli olduğu öngörüldü.
b. Yapılan konferansta palyatif tıp (hafifletici, destekleyici tedavi) yöntemlerinin yaygınlık kazanmasının gerekli olduğu öngörüldü.
c. EN 'It has been foreseen in the conference that the spread of palliative medical methods is essential.'

Sentences (13a) and (13b) both include a borrowed expression *palyatif tıp* (EN 'palliative medicine') which does not have an exact literal equivalent in Turkish. Sentence (13b) includes the borrowed expression with a brief explanation *hafifletici, destekleyici tedavi* (EN 'mitigating', 'supportive treatment'). 83.6% of respondents found sentence (13b) clearer. As the decision-maker, the translator could explain a borrowed term which is not generally known by the public briefly in order to render the text in a functional way in line with the aim of the target text.

In the last question, I compared the understandability of new coinages in Turkish and borrowed terms.

(14) a. Katarakt, göz sorunlarının en yaygın görülen şeklidir. Bunun için düzenli kontrollerinizi yaptırın.
b. Akbasma, göz sorunlarının en yaygın görülen şeklidir. Bunun için düzenli kontrollerinizi yaptırın.
c. EN 'Cataracts is the most common eye defect. Therefore, you should visit your doctor for regular check-ups.'

Sentence (14a) includes an older borrowed term as *katarakt* (EN 'cataracts'). However, sentence (14b) includes the literal equivalent of the borrowed term *(akbasma)*, which is newly coined in Turkish. 68.9% of respondents found sentence (14a) clearer. Based on this observation, it will be appropriate to say that borrowed expressions could be more transparent than literal equivalents on the condition that the borrowed expression is older and more acceptable than the literal derivation. Therefore, we can say that the perception of the readership is the main determinant for the functioning of the translated term into the target system.

6 Conclusion

Popular medical texts serve as informative texts and they are written to inform individuals from various segments of society about trendy topics in health issues, news, diseases, and innovations in medicine. Therefore, the main aim of popular medical translations is to transfer the message and the relevant content to the target readership in a transparent and understandable way. As the comprehension of the translation is closely related to the understanding of the words or terms used in the text, it is expected from the translator to take appropriate decisions within the process of translating and to follow the proper procedures as per the requirements of the target society. For instance, translators could make some predictions on the basis of their observations about the attitudes, expectations and reading habits of target readers. Popular medical texts are accessible to a large number of individuals via magazines, internet, newspapers or brochures and using transparent terms in the target text plays a crucial role in the comprehension of the text by a broad readership.

When the corpus study is considered, it is observed that borrowing (63.4%) is the most widely chosen translation procedure in translating one-word terms in popular medical texts. Most borrowings include naturalisation, that is to say, the words are borrowed from English, but adapted to Turkish grammatical and morphological rules. Borrowing is followed by literal translation (30.7%) which is realized by choosing the literal equivalent of the word from the Turkish lexicon. Other procedures are rarely used.

Unlike one-word terms, hybrid combinations are generally used for the translations of multi-word terms. The procedures of borrowing and literal translation are generally used together in the translation of multi-word terms. Borrowing-literal combination is followed by multi-word terms translated just literally; and borrowing is the third most widely-used method for multi-word terms. In other words, procedures chosen for the translation of one-word terms and multi-word terms differ.

It is the translator's task to determine the aim of the target text (which is here transferring the message in an acceptable and understandable way to the target audience) and to choose the most appropriate methods within the translation process. While choosing the procedure of borrowing for translation of terms in popular medical texts, the translator should pay attention to the transparency level of the term for target readers.

Some borrowings could be easily understood by medical staff, but lead to confusion on the minds of target readers. Using unfamiliar borrowings makes the target text non-transparent. As seen from the survey results, target readers do not perceive borrowings as transparent expressions that they have not heard before. The procedure of borrowing could be used to the extent that the borrowed term is welcomed and truly understood by target readers, that is to say, borrowing may be the appropriate procedure if the borrowed term has become an accepted element of the target language. If not, literal translation could be chosen instead of borrowings.

If literal translation of a term does not make sense to the readership and feels awkward, other methods in harmony with the target potential could be used. Transposition, modulation or equivalence are some of the methods that could be applied in that case.

If there is no solution except for borrowing (for example there is no understandable literal equivalent), the borrowed expression could be explained in order to be transparent for target laymen. Using an explanation is acceptable for the translation of popular medical texts, the aim of which is to render the message to target readers in a transparent, concise and coherent way. Translation of terms in an understandable way will also arouse curiosity among target readers for popular medical texts. Therefore, medical information reaches large masses and the information becomes more accessible and applicable by individuals.

References

Ammann, Margret (2008), *Akademik Çeviri Eğitimine Giriş,* Ekeman, E. Deniz (trans.), Istanbul: Multilingual.

BBC News (2014), 'Organ transplants: 'Supercooling' keeps organs fresh', http://www.bbc.com/news/health-28061265 (viewed 17 Sept. 2014).

BBC Türkçe (2014), 'Derin soğutma nakil öncesi organ ömrünü uzatabilir', http://www.bbc.co.uk/turkce/haberler/2014/06/140630_organ_nakli_derin_sogutma (viewed 17 Sept. 2014).

Collins Dictionary (2014), 'Anaerobic', http://www.collinsdictionary.com/dictionary/english/anaerobic (viewed 17 Sept. 2014).

Dirckx, John H. (2006), 'Greek and Latin in Medical Terminology', in Stegman, Julie K.; Branger, Eric; Piper, Tiffany; Filardo, Thomas W.; Dirckx, John H.; Lukens, Raymond & Hensyl, William R. (eds.), *Stedman's Medical Dictionary*, 28th ed., Philadelphia: Lippincott Williams & Wilkins, appendix 9, downloadable from http://stedmansonline.com/webFiles/Dict-Stedmans28/APP04.pdf (downloaded 1 March 2015).

Finkenstaedt, Thomas & Wolff, Dieter (1973), *Ordered profusion; studies in dictionaries and the English lexicon*, Heidelberg: C. Winter.

Herget, Katrin & Alegre, Teresa (2009), 'Translation of Medical Terms', *Translation Journal* 13 (3), http://www.translationjournal.net/journal/49medical1.htm (viewed 17 Sept. 2014).

Löning, Petra (1981), 'Zur medizinischen Fachsprache. Stilistische Gliederung und Textanalysen', *Muttersprache* 91:79-92.

Munday, Jeremy (2008), *Introducing Translation Studies: Theories and Applications,* London: Routledge.

Newmark, Peter (1988), *A Textbook of Translation,* New York: Prentice-Hall International.

Pearson, Jennifer (1998), *Terms in Context*, Amsterdam/Philadelphia: John Benjamins Publishing.

Pym, Anthony (2010), *Exploring Translation Theories,* London: Routledge.

Radu, Mirela (2008), 'English for Medical Purpose Teaching', *Romanian Journal of Stomatology, LIV*(2-3): 145-147.

Reiss, Katharina (2000), *Translation Criticism: The Potentials and Limitations,* Rhodes, Erroll F. (trans.), Manchester, UK: St. Jerome Publishing.

Reiss, Katharina & Vermeer, Hans J. (1984), *Grundlegung einer allgemeinen Translationstheorie*, Tübingen: Niemeyer.

Toury, Gideon (1995), *Descriptive Translation Studies – and beyond,* Amsterdam/Philadelphia: John Benjamins Publishing Company.

Wikipedia (2014), 'Latin influence in English', http://en.wikipedia.org/wiki/Latin_influence_in_English (viewed 17 Sept. 2014).

Vermeer, Hans J. (2000), 'Skopos and Commission in Translational Action', in Venuti, Lawrence (ed.), *The Translation Studies Reader*, London and New York: Routledge, pp. 221–32.

Vinay, Jean-Paul & Darbelnet, Jean (1995), *Comparative Stylistics of French and English,* Sager, Juan C. & Hamel, Marie-Josée (trans. and eds.), Amsterdam: John Benjamins Publishing Company.

CHAPTER SEVEN

COMPRESSION AS A FACTOR BEHIND THE BORROWING OF ENGLISH MEDICAL TERMINOLOGY INTO POLISH

MARIUSZ GÓRNICZ

Differences between terms that are brought to light when terminological systems of the same domain in two or more natural languages are compared are due to a number of causes, the most important of which is incompatibility (asymmetry) between concept systems and differences in language systems that influence the inventory of term formation models available for use in the respective languages.

These factors can be construed as being related to the plane of content or to the plane of expression. Plane-of-content differences may stem from insufficient development of the domain in one language or from differences in concept systems. The former situation is frequently seen when there exists a culture or language where a particular domain is more developed (such as the Italian language with regard to classical music); such gaps are also continually closed, e.g. via the borrowing of terms. Differences between concept systems also occur in domains whose concept systems are country-specific, as is the case with legal terminology, which is informed by a variety of legal traditions (e.g. Roman law vs. common law) and may also reflect different social policies or ideological influences (cf. narcotic laws in different countries or the penalisation of particular political views). Unlike such asymmetrical systems, symmetrical ones, including terminologies of various branches of science, are – ideally – characterized by a one-to-one correspondence between concept systems. Importantly, this correspondence pertains to terms with their underlying concepts in different languages. Differences between different schools of thought within a science are not considered here.

The concept system of medicine is symmetrical within the so-called Western medicine paradigm. Other paradigms, for example, that of

Tibetan medicine, are usually vastly different. Even though they embrace the same reality of symptoms and treatments, behind seemingly similar conceptualisations at the observational level are incompatible higher-level concepts.

Practitioners of Tibetan medicine distinguish three types of abnormal urine appearance (cf. amchikunga.com, no date). Each type may be mapped to particular abnormalities recognised by Western medicine. However, the observational level is where the similarity begins and ends as Tibetan medicine ascribes these abnormalities to disorders of wind, bile and phlegm, respectively. Wind, bile and phlegm disorders affect many other organs and do not tally with groupings of conditions known to Western medicine.[1] Apparent or partial correspondence at this lowest level of a conceptual system thus need not entail identity at higher tiers.

1 Symmetry and asymmetry in medical terminology

Symmetry between terminological systems of medicine in different language communities is greatly aided by the presence of Latin and Greek combining forms. Terms made up of such stems are easily reproducible in other languages owing to shared combinatorial rules. Sets of Graeco-Latin (i.e. Neoclassical) stems are called *terminological keys* [orig. *Terminologieschlüssel* (Felber, Budin 1989:131)] and are domain-specific. They may reflect the current scientific paradigm, particularly if they are the dominant term formation method. For example, in medicine, the use of the prefixes *hypo-* and *hyper-* as combining forms reflects the belief that a deficit or excess of particular substances in the body can lead to disease.

While such combining forms are formally borrowings from Latin and Greek, they often "go unnoticed as borrowings" (Cabré 1999: 89). In the Polish linguistic tradition, they are called "artificial borrowings" (Jadacka 1999: 1773), which perhaps aptly reflects the fact that Latin and Greek combining forms are used to form new terms in contemporary languages while the languages they derive from are extinct.

Similar to the creation of composite terms comprising two or more combining forms used as stems is the use of complex words derived from Latin and formed by the addition of affixal morphemes to single stems, as in *infection* or *decortication.* Polish medical terminology includes a number of similar affixal derivatives (*za-każ-enie* [perfective prefix +

[1] Here the term *Western medicine* is used to refer to 'mainstream' evidence-based medicine of today. It does not include alternative medicine (homoeopathy, etc.) or ancient Greek medicine.

blight + gerundive suffix, '*infection*'], *od-wodni-enie* [*de* + *water* + gerundive suffix, '*dehydration*']), with some representing calques of their Latin equivalents (*od-wodni-enie – de-hydr-ation*).

Medical eponyms constitute another category of medical terms shared between languages. Some eponymic terms are reproduced in a number of languages, while others are modified. The result can be an eponym with different names, e.g. *Crohn's disease* vs. *choroba Leśniowskiego-Crohna* ('Leśniowski-Crohn disease') in Polish, or a non-eponymic term may be used instead. As an illustration of the latter, Russian *болезнь Боткина* [bolezn' Botkina] 'Botkin's disease' used to be the standard term for viral hepatitis and the Polish equivalent of *Hodgkin's lymphoma* is *ziarnica złośliwa* ('malignant granulomatosis').

Differences between the form of equivalent terms in different languages may be due to the use of different methods of term formation (e.g. creating multi-word terms vs. composition as in the case of EN *hormone therapy* vs. PL *hormonoterapia*), the choice of terms that reflect different aspects of the concept they denote, or the choice of terms representing different levels of transparency.

Aspectual synonyms are terms that describe the same concept from different perspectives. By way of example, the disease *infectious mononucleosis* has also been known as all four of the names in (1).

(1)
a. monocytic angina
b. glandular fever
c. Pfeiffer's disease
d. kissing disease

The names in (1) refer to different aspects of this medical condition: inflammation of the pharynx and the presence of mononuclear cells in the blood (1a); elevated temperature and lymph node enlargement (1b); the author of an early description (1c); and a characteristic mode of transmission (1d).

An important division of terms in general is that of analytical and non-analytical terms. Analytical terms are those made up wholly of words or word elements that possess only specialised meanings (Musiołek-Choiński 1986: 50-56) and refer to salient aspects of the definition of the concept corresponding to the term. Salient aspects of a concept are those present in its Aristotelian intensional definition (*per genus proximum et differentia specifica*). Non-analytical terms contain at least one element that does not correspond to a salient aspect of the concept and include eponymic terms, terms incorporating symbols (*vitamin A*) and metaphorical/metonymic terms, which merit further subdivision and a comment.

Metaphorical adjectives derived from language for general purposes (LGP), such as *early* or *cold*, commonly accompany headwords in multi-word terms. They refer to scalable qualities and while they may mean different points on their respective scales in different terms (*early-onset coronary heart disease* occurs before the age of 55-60 years, but *early-onset diabetes* is a synonym for *type 1 diabetes mellitus* and occurs in children), they need to be set apart from metaphorical terms where the metaphor is unique, such as *shaggy pericardium, whistling face syndrome, cri du chat syndrome*. Metaphors of this kind often accompany such general terms as *disease* or *syndrome*. Terms in this group are metonymic as well as metaphorical, since the metaphor usually points to a manifestation of the disease.

Such metaphorical terms are generally unique since the metaphorical components do not indicate the place of the underlying concept in the concept system and so they normally do not easily collocate with other headwords. They are also relatively short as, being non-hierarchical, they do not give rise to subordinate terms. Terms incorporating a scalable adjective are in between analytical and non-analytical term groups.

2 Terminological compression

Compression (condensation) has a wide meaning in linguistics and many representations in language, beginning with the use of non-finite verb forms when the context clarifies what finite elements the verb is carrying: the participle in *standing on the platform* is understood to represent third person plural past tense in the sentence *The people standing on the platform didn't see anything*. In another example: *We forced him to obey*, the pronoun *him* is the object of the main clause verb *force*, which is a control verb, but it also indicates the subject of the verb *obey* (EJO 1999:308). Syntactic condensation often involves using non-finite verb forms instead of subordinate clauses. It may lead to ambiguity: *Jack is tired of the gossiping* may mean 'he is tired of being gossiped about' or 'he is tired of gossiping about others'.

Another example of condensation in language is the particular use of deverbal nouns that has come to be known as *grammatical metaphor*. Grammatical metaphor "operates primarily by turning clauses into nouns; that is, by replacing clauses with nominal groups" (Guillén Galve 1998:369). As Halliday (1994:352) puts it, "By this device, processes (...) and properties (...) are reworded metaphorically as nouns; instead of functioning in the clause, as Process or Attribute, they function as Thing in the nominal group". What is left out is the time reference, which can, however, be recovered on the basis of article use in English, as illustrated in (2).

(2) a. If nerve penetration occurs ('If a nerve **is** penetrated')
b. As a result of (the) nerve penetration… ('As the nerve **was** penetrated during the procedure')

In (2a), the nominalization has a generic interpretation, referring to any instance of nerve penetration, as indicated by the absence of an article. The definite article in (2b) suggests that the reference is to a specific event, i.e. an event of nerve penetration taking place at a particular time.

The essence of lexical compression is well exemplified by the use of adjectives. In LDOCE (2003:506), the adjective *electric* has the following meanings: "1. Needing electricity to work, produced by electricity, or used for carrying electricity (*electric light/kettle/cooker/current/power/charge*); 2. Making people feel very excited." The second meaning is not relevant to our purposes since it is a derived, metaphorical one, but the first one, which might be summarised as 'related to electricity', is made up of a range of senses which are brought to light when individual compounds are analysed. These finer distinctions, exemplified by collocations such as *electric kettle, electric light* and *electric cable*, usually go unnoticed since language users are able to fill in the missing information regarding the exact nature of the relation between electricity and the object denoted by the head noun by reflecting on the characteristics of the concept. For example, language users interpret the meaning of *electric* in *electric kettle* as 'indicating the source of energy for heating the water' because they realize that a kettle is used for boiling water rather than supplying energy and that an act of boiling water necessitates a supply of energy. That, however, is left out of the lexical structure of this noun phrase – and that is compression.

In terminology, the concept of compression refers to the condensation of a term's surface structure relative to its conceptual content (Leitchik 1981, Musiołek-Choiński 1986:143-150, Górnicz 1997, STP 2005:50). Terminological compression serves to produce shorter terms at the expense of transparency or explicitness. "A term or appellation is considered transparent when the concept it designates can be inferred, at least partially, without a definition or an explanation. In other words, the meaning of a term or appellation can be deduced from its parts" (ISO-704 2009:39). A transparent term is thus one whose lexical meaning (LM, that produced by combining the identifiable meanings of all components) is close to or identical with the conceptual or terminological meaning (TM, as given by the definition). Consequently, the ultimate transparent term is the defining part of a definition (i.e. *definiens*). Obviously, such long terms would be quite cumbersome to use; hence the need for condensing the conceptual content in the plane of expression.

The terms in (3) describe the heart condition characterised by pain in the chest at times of insufficient blood supply to a part of the heart muscle due to narrowing of one or more coronary arteries differ in the degree of compression.

(3) a. ischaemic heart disease (IHD)
b. coronary heart disease
c. angina pectoris
d. dławica piersiowa [‘choking-disease chest$_{ADJ}$’, i.e. chest-choking condition]
e. dusznica bolesna [‘shortness-of-breath-disease painful’, i.e.painful shortness-of-breath condition].
f. stenocardia

(3a) is a typical analytical term profiling the site of the disease and the cause of the problem (ischaemia, or inadequate blood supply). (3b) is less transparent as it only indicates that the disease affects the heart and, more specifically, the coronary vessels within the heart. (3c) is an older term that points to a choking sensation (angina) and the chest as the site of the problem, and so do its Polish equivalents (3d) and (3e). As is the rule with Polish terms, the head nouns are the left-most elements, being followed by their adjective modifiers. (3c), (3d) and (3e) do not refer to the cause. Currently, they are used to name the hallmark symptom of IHD. Finally, the Latinate compound (3f) refers to the heart as the site of the problem and to narrowing as the cause. However, it is not supposed to mean ‘narrowing of the heart’.

The concept of transparency is about comparing the formal meanings of a term’s components to the intension of the underlying concept as expressed by the definition. The definition itself is assumed to be known and well-established. Such situations need to be distinguished from cases when the definition is not clear, i.e. when the concept is being formed. In such cases, the semantic transparency of a particular container (i.e. term) is not important as there is pragmatic opacity (the underlying concept is not clear to the users).

3 Techniques of terminological compression

The following presentation of techniques of term compression is based on Leitchik (1981) with some modifications (Górnicz 1997). Term compression may be achieved in a number of ways:

- Phonetic simplification: simplifying the pronunciation (and spelling) of a term by eliding or replacing segments or syllables. Phonetic compression occurs in individual words. The presence of lipids in the blood is denoted by a composite of the combining forms *lipid-* and *-aemia* for blood, thus *lipidaemia*. However, it is normally shortened to *lipaemia*. The stem denoting lipids is still recognizable and the omitted segment (*id*) is not meaningful within this stem; thus, there is only phonetic change.

- Derivational compression consists in forming a complex or compound word to replace a multi-word term or a part of it. It may also be called univerbation. Lexical vagueness and the distance from the terminological meaning often increase as the suffix often does not precisely indicate the generic concept. For example, the suffix *-oma* refers mostly to neoplastic growths, but is also found in names of conditions that are not tumours, such as *haematoma* ('bruise').

- Morphological compression (Leitchik 1981:71) involves the use of 'false morphemes' obtained by an etymologically 'illegal' division of a word, as when *hamburger* was split into *ham+burger* and the new 'morpheme' was subsequently used to form names for similar dishes (*cheeseburger)*. A more serious example in terminology is the suffix *-on* denoting elementary particles in physics (originally from the indivisible word *electron*, subsequently used to form such terms as *prot+on, neutr+on*, etc.). Blending (*smoke+fog* ⇒ *smog*) is also regarded as morphological compression.

- Semantic compression consists in removing words corresponding to certain components of the concept from the term. It is illustrated in (4).

(4) a. wrzodziejące zapalenie jelita grubego
[ulcerative inflammation of the large intestine] ('ulcerative colitis')

b. krwotoczne zapalenie jelita grubego
[haemorrhagic inflammation of the large intestine]
('haemorrhagic colitis')

c. wrzodziejąco-krwotoczne zapalenie jelita grubego
[ulcerative-haemorrhagic inflammation of the large intestine]
('ulcerative-haemorrhagic colitis')

The Polish expressions in (4) have the same meaning. (4c) expresses this by a combination of adjectives of which one is not present in (4a) and (4b). Therefore, (4a) and (4b) represent semantic compression compared to the more complete (4c). The most frequently used term is (4a), although it is not the most transparent one.

- Liaison compression is a type of semantic compression where the elements omitted represent semantic links between the remaining elements of a compound term. As a result, the lexical meaning of the term is null. The term *coronary heart disease* involves liaison compression since the information that the adjective *coronary* refers to the coronary arteries of the heart cannot be retrieved from the form of the term. The conceptual linkage between this element and the rest of the term is clear only to those who are familiar with the underlying concept. Similarly, *optic neuritis* is inflammation of the optic nerve, while combinatorial analysis of the lexical meaning might suggest that it is an optic type of nerve inflammation. Liaison compression leads to the creation of short terms that are intelligible only to specialists in the field, who can supply the components of the definition conveyed by the omitted elements.

- Metonymy/metaphor: metonymic terms focus on secondary features of the concept. Metonymy may be called radical semantic compression. Such secondary features may not be included in the definition. Metaphorical terms profile similarity between the concept in question and a concept from another domain. Such similarity is not contained in the definition of the original concept. The term *sunset sign* associates a particular manner of eyeball positioning with a natural phenomenon. *Kissing ulcers* refers to a pair of ulcers found on opposite surfaces of the gastric mucosa.

Metaphorical/metonymic terms fail to comply with a number of term formation principles, e.g. they are not transparent and do not point to the position of the concept within the relevant concept system. However, they often denote concepts where an analytical term would not be possible. It would, for example, be rather difficult to develop a system of topographic analytical terms to describe the position of the eyeballs in various conditions.

Metonymic/metaphorical terms where the head word is a general medical term (*sign/symptom, disease/syndrome*, etc.) and the metaphorical element is the modifier should be distinguished from those (often used in texts in the form of single words) where the head word is non-terminological, i.e. has been derived from LGP. Such terms are the result of semantic derivation (semasiological term formation, ten Hacken 2008: 985), which consists in refining (usually narrowing) the meaning of a general language word, as in the computer science term *memory.* However, an LGP word may enter terminology as a metaphorical term, as is the case with *computer mouse*, or *head* and *tail* when used to describe the structure of a viral particle, as these terms only have physical similarity in common with the original word.

- Eponymic terms are also metonymic, substituting the name of the discoverer (or patient) of a particular disease, anatomical structure or treatment method for the disease, structure or method (*listeriosis, duct of Wirsung, Hartnup disease*). Eponymic terms possess very low transparency as the names so commemorated are hardly ever significant for the concepts (in the case of discoverers) or lose their currency over time (*Lou Gehrig's disease*).

- Semiotic compression refers to the formation of terms incorporating symbols, as in *α particle.* Isolated terms exhibiting this type of compression are not transparent, but families of terms including the same symbol in the same meaning are more meaningful, as in *α particle, α radiation, α decay.* Numbers are also commonly used to form semiotically compressed terms, e.g. *interleukin 1, 2,* etc.

Terms containing symbols are a way to avoid the problem of using a term whose lexical meaning is not compatible with the conceptual meaning. Many of the compounds now known as *interleukin 1..., interleukin 17* used to have a number of names. Interleukin 8 used to be known under more than 10 names, highlighting different functions (genenames.org 2014). These functions were not initially linked to the same compound. When it was finally realised that one molecule was responsible for all these effects, it was clear that no name in use reflected even a few of those functions, and the use of a semiotically compressed term, or a similar lexically near-empty form, was quite advisable.

- Abbreviation: the use of abbreviations and acronyms is discussed as the last type of term compression since an abbreviation never stands alone, always complementing a full form of the term. Isolated abbreviations are not transparent on their own, but families of abbreviations may make their members transparent. The elements of abbreviations shared by all members of a family actually represent "false morphemes". An acronymic family once formed of names of car factories in the Soviet Union (*ZAZ, UAZ, BelAZ*), where the initial component referred to the town that housed the factory and the last two letters stood for 'car factory' (автомобильный завод, [*avtomobil'nyj zavod*]) (Ickovich 1972).

Interestingly, the authors of major textbooks or manuals on terminology do not directly describe terminological compression, although they often refer to its consequences. Felber & Budin (1989:121) write about the "degree of abbreviation" of the description of a concept, stating that a multi-word term (*Maschine zum Hobeln* 'machine for planing') represents either a full description of a concept or a minor condensation of the conceptual content, a compound term (*Hobelmaschine* 'planing machine') represents a major condensation of concept description and a derivative (*Hobler* 'planer') is the shortest possible combination of elements. The shorter a name is, the greater its polysemy: *Hobler* may refer to a tool or to someone who uses that tool.

Sager (1990: 66) notes that "there is a tendency to reduce longer compounds to their shortest possible forms: (...) *magazine feeding attachment -> magazine feed -> magazine*; *power-operated feed -> power feed*." He states that "an originally free collocation, e.g. *a box for tools*, can be reduced step by step to its shortest form, e.g. *tool box*, *tool-box*, *toolbox*.", noting the brevity of such terms as well as their lack of transparency: "e.g. *diamond drilling* signifies drilling by means of diamond drill bits, whereas *concrete drilling* signifies drilling into concrete."

Gilreath (1995: 34) notes that eponyms and term-ordinal hybrids (e.g., *concept-3*) "may be precise but non-transparent", and this statement reflects the distinction between the terminological meaning and lexical meaning of a term.

Finally, ten Hacken (this volume) mentions as a source of opacity of terms that the meaning of a compound is determined in part by the relation between the two components, but this relation is not specified in the expression. This description clearly corresponds to liaison compression as defined above. Accordingly, it appears advisable to bring the concept of terminological compression to the attention of the community of terminologists and lexicologists as this should facilitate the description and interpretation of certain phenomena in term formation.

Table 7-1 gives an overview of compression techniques. The table headings carry the implication that a non-analytical term is in some way inferior to an analytical one or that analytical terms are primary to non-analytical ones. The question arises now whether metaphorical nomination in terminology actually ought to be regarded as a secondary rather than primary naming technique. The answer lies in the defining features of science and scientific terminology. Science is supposed to describe the world in an objective manner and so the vehicles of this description, i.e. terms, ought to be precise, objective and impartial. The requirement of precision, understood as the existence of a clear link between a term and its associated concept, is not compatible with most non-analytical terms, which, as the examples given above show, fail to capture the most salient characteristics of the concept they denote. That is their main weakness: they fail to comply with some important principles of term formation; most importantly, the one of logicality, i.e. denoting the place of a concept in the relevant concept system.

Techniques of terminological compression leading to:	
A new analytical term	A non-analytical term
Phonetic simplification	Metaphoric/metonymic compression
Derivational compression	Eponymic compression
Morphological compression	Semiotic compression
Semantic compression	Liaison compression
Abbreviation	

Table 7-1. Division of techniques of terminological compression

Another principle of term formation is monosemy. Monosemy is a prerequisite of objectivity and a metaphorical term is by definition polysemous, containing a reference to an object from another domain, which may weigh on the semantic interpretation of the term.

Thus, the principle of objective description (and terminological representation) of salient features of the world's objects and phenomena, coupled with the requirement of monosemy, provides the rationale for considering metaphorical terms a type of compression vis-à-vis their analytical equivalents.

4 Polish equivalents of English metaphorical terms

Early medical terminology in Greek and Latin relied on metaphor. The Greek word καρκίνος [karkinos], and its Latin translation *cancer*, originally meant 'crab, crayfish'. Hippocrates used it to refer to indurated tumours on the basis of physical resemblance (Zieliński 2004:125). The *gastrocnemius*, the muscle which gives the calf a convex shape, includes the stem *gastro-*, referring to the stomach. An example of an early medical term representing a metaphor in Polish is *komora* ('cardiac or cerebral ventricle'), the primary meaning of which was 'a room without a furnace, a chamber'.

Today metaphorical terms which contain LGP lexis, including colloquial vocabulary are still being added to English medical terminology, but their established Polish equivalents are often analytical. When the Polish equivalent is a calque, it is often accompanied in texts by signals of its alien status, such as being placed in quotation marks or preceded by qualifying phrases such as *tzw.* ['so-called']. Not uncommonly, such terms are also borrowed.

It appears that the use vs. non-use of metaphorical terms or, more broadly, of LGP words is a characteristic feature of national (country-specific) terminologies. The examples shown in the following part of the article seem to indicate that Polish users of medical terminology are rather unwilling to accept such terms, even though the linguistic means for reproducing them (by calquing) are available and there are no grammatical restrictions.

To illustrate the above, I will use examples from a variety of sources, including original contributions in orthopaedics and rehabilitation submitted to the journal *Ortopedia Traumatologia Rehabilitacja* (http:// www.ortopedia.com.pl). Each issue of the journal includes approximately 10 contributions originally written in Polish, which brings the total number of texts from this source reviewed in search of borrowings (2007 – present) to approximately 500 texts of 8-10 pages each.

Click probably ranks among the best known technolectal borrowings from English, second only to the likes of *computer*, *video* and others, which predated it. In Polish, the verb has been assimilated to *kliknąć*, and the noun is a derivative of the verb (*kliknięcie*). The LGP meaning of *click* conceptualises a sound, while the LSP meaning conceptualises an activity or its result. The sound is a secondary feature of the technical act of pressing a mouse button. *Click* is thus precisely a metonymic (ATTRIBUTE FOR ACTIVITY), rather than metaphorical, term. The borrowing of this verb may have been due to its non-analytical nature. It has to be admitted, though, that there is no verb in Polish that would correspond to *click* in all of its many meanings, as indicated in (5).

(5) a. click one's tongue ('<u>cmoknąć</u> językiem z irytacją')
b. click one's fingers ('<u>pstryknąć</u> palcami')
c. click one's heels ('<u>stuknąć</u> obcasami')

The three senses in (5) are all translated using different verbs (underlined) and (5a) also contains an adverbial of manner (*z irytacją* 'with irritation'). *Click* is also a term in phonetics denoting a type of ingressive sound, and its Polish equivalent *mlask* did find its way into some computer manuals in the early 1990s, but this use did not survive, most probably because of undesirable associations with the verb *mlaskać* ('eat noisily, smack one's lips').

The word *kinking* is a medical term in cardiology referring to a sharp bend in an artery (coronary or other) that makes it difficult to insert a catheter, impedes blood flow through that artery, etc. Outside terminology, it is the gerundial form of the verb *to kink,* of which the zero-derived nominal form has the following meanings „1. a twist in something that is normally straight; 2. a small problem in a plan, system, etc.; 3. something strange or dangerous in someone's character" (LDOCE 2003:888). The terminological meaning is based on the most common LGP meaning. In Polish, this term is obviously completely non-transparent, and its proper use requires memorising the definition. However, it is quite well-established in medical Polish: it is declined (*kinking-kinkingu*, etc.) just like many other borrowings with the suffix *-ing*, and it has also been used in article titles, e.g. in a 2004 report titled "Kinking tętnicy szyjnej wewnętrznej – ocena występowania…" ['Kinking of internal carotid artery – actual incidence…'] (Madycki *et al.* 2004). In the body of the article, the author alternated between *kinking* and the analytical indigenous term *zagięcie kątowe* (bend$_{N}$ angular, 'angular bend').

The next example is *gate control theory*, sometimes abbreviated to *gate theory*, which refers to a theory that postulates that the conduction of pain stimuli across certain nerve fibres in the spinal cord is stifled when certain other fibres are stimulated. Devices for electrical nerve stimulation supposed to produce pain control, e.g. in back pain sufferers, are based on this theoretical premise. The use of the word *gate* makes the English term metaphorical and non-transparent, while also contributing to its pragmatic function: a prospective buyer of a pain-control device will find it easier to remember the principle being put to use in the device by remembering the metaphorical gate which controls the passage of pain stimuli.

Several years ago, the Polish equivalent was *teoria kontrolowanego przepustu rdzeniowego* ('theory controlled$_{GEN}$ throughput$_{GEN}$ medullary$_{GEN}$', i.e. theory of controlled medullary throughput). The Polish term is a typical analytical formation made up of three components associated with the language of medicine/science (*teoria, przepust, rdzeniowy*) and one component known to LGP users and used in a partly metaphorical sense (*kontrolowany*).

In more recent texts, one may find Polish equivalents that are more formally similar to the English term, e.g. *teoria bramki kontrolnej* (lit. 'theory of gate controlling$_{ADJ}$', i.e. control gate theory), *teoria bramki bólu/bólowej* (lit. 'theory of gate of pain$_{N/ADJ}$', i.e. pain gate theory) or *teoria bramkowania* (lit. 'theory of gating', i.e. gating theory). It is important to note that *gate* has been rendered in these equivalents not as the LGP word *brama* or *furtka*, but as the diminutive *bramka*, which is actually a term in logic (*bramka logiczna*, lit. 'gate logical', i.e. logic gate) and in electronics (*bramka*, 'gate'), as a component of a particular type of transistor). It also happens to be the word for *goal* in football. It should therefore be described as a metaphorical borrowing from another LSP concept field rather than from LGP. Note that, in the equivalents above, the word *bramka* is also always qualified by a post-posed adjective (*kontrolna, bólowa*), which makes it look term-like in a similar manner as the pre-posed modifier in *gate control theory* makes it look term-like. In multi-word terms in Polish containing adjectives, the adjectives are normally placed to the right of the head noun. *Bramkowanie*, in turn, is a gerundive form that is not found in LGP. Overall, these examples indicate that while there may be a trend towards metaphorical naming in Polish term formation patterns, the Polish equivalents still carry more academic pretence compared to the original English terms.

A similar trend can be seen with *złamanie podokostnowe* (fracture$_N$ subperiosteal$_{ADJ}$. 'subperiosteal fracture'), which is a type of fracture that does not disrupt the contour of the fractured bone. In English it is popularly termed *greenstick fracture* by virtue of a similarity between the appearance of this kind of fracture in a radiographic image and the appearance of a broken young twig, which bends but does not break. Non-analytical Polish equivalents emulating the original metaphorical term also exist, but note that along with the nearly word-for-word equivalent *złamanie zielonej gałązki* ('fracture of green twig'), there is *złamanie "zielonej gałązki"*, with the quotation marks signalling alienness interpretable as incompatibility with common term formation patterns, and *złamanie typu zielonej gałązki* ('fracture of the green twig type'), with the addition of the word *type* possibly in an attempt to make it sound more academic.

Natural killers, or *natural killer cells*, sometimes abbreviated to *NK cells*, is the name of certain immune cells that are capable of destroying other cells, e.g. cancer cells, without first being activated by so-called antigen presenting cells. The only widely accepted Polish equivalent is *komórki NK* ('cells NK'), suggesting again that a more metaphorical rendition is not acceptable. The abbreviation at least does not carry undesirable connotations. Interestingly, in Russian, *натуральные киллеры* ([*naturalnyje killery*] *'natural killers')* is the established form. It has given rise to the derivative *киллерные клетки* ([*killernyje kletki*] 'killer$_{ADJ}$ cells'). This example shows that attitudes to metaphorical terms may differ between speakers of related languages, apparently giving more credence to the statement that such differences are a pragmatic rather than intralinguistic phenomenon.

Czas przeżycia endoprotez (lit. 'time of survival of implants', i.e. implant survival time) is another example of a term including metaphorical content. *Survival* reflects the metaphor MEDICAL DEVICE IS LIVING BEING. In the Polish texts, the term was preceded by *tzw.* or the word *przeżycia* ('survival') was placed in quotation marks. Another Polish term is also used: *żywotność endoprotezy* (lit. 'viability of implant'. i.e. 'implant viability'). It is less metaphorical since there is a tradition of using the word *żywotność* with regard to inanimate objects, such as materials. It was less often used in the texts I have studied. A recently attested equivalent is *biofunkcjonalność* ('biofunctionality'), which might be interpreted as indicating a trend of moving away from calquing metaphorical terms and towards using analytical equivalents.

The two sentence fragments in (6) show that even words free from logic-defying metaphorical shifts may be regarded as alien.

(6) a. uszkodzenia chrząstki stawowej o charakterze uskoku (schodka;ang. step)
[lesions of articular cartilage of the fault (step; Eng. step) type],
b. drugi określa wielkość uszkodzenia o charakterze przerwy (ang. gap)
[the other defines the extent of a lesion of the gap (Eng. gap) type].

In (6a), the Polish equivalent given in brackets is the dictionary equivalent of 'step' and the equivalent given before the brackets (*uskok*, 'fault') is a term used in geology to denote a tectonic fracture of a volume of rock. The author thus opts for a transtechnolectal metaphor rather than using an LGP word even though the latter's semantic constraints apparently do not clash with the new usage, quite unlike the case of *implant survival*. In (6b), the provision of the original term in brackets may be interpreted as a safeguard against possible criticism of the use of a word that is not primarily a term, although the use of this word to denote an empty space between two bone fragments is also not particularly eyebrow-raising. The addition of the equivalent in brackets is probably not related to the author wishing to quote the division of cartilage lesions in the original since more complete terms (*step lesion*, *gap lesion*) were not quoted.

5 Equivalents of terms exhibiting liaison compression

The term *in-out-in technique*, which describes a technique for stabilizing fractures with a screw that pierces cortical bone, has been rendered as *technika "in-out-in"*. The lexical (combinatorial) meaning of this term amounts to almost nil, since we might speculate that the technique, i.e. procedure, in question involves introducing, then removing, then reinserting an instrument, but otherwise are left wondering about the details.

The presence of the borrowing in the Polish term may just reflect this lack of semantic liaison within the term or result from the grammatical impossibility of using prepositions as noun modifiers in Polish (e.g. *on-off switch* vs *przycisk włącz-wyłącz* [lit. 'button switch on-switch off', with the head noun followed by the modifier]).[2]

It should be added at this point that some terms representing liaison compression have survived in Polish medical terminology, including the equivalents of *coronary heart disease* and *stenocardia*, as discussed earlier on. Latinate terms are especially prone to various types of compression, attempting as they do to portray a concept with usually just two meaningful components. Let us also note that some time-honoured Latinate terms have lexical meanings that are plainly wrong when set beside the underlying concept. *Anaemia*, for one, does not denote lack of blood even though it is broken down etymologically into *an-* 'absence of sth, no' and *-aemia* 'blood'. *Leukaemia*, in turn, can only be regarded as fairly analytical when we assume that *leuk-* means 'leukocyte' here, rather than 'white', a meaning that it has in *leukoplakia*.

6 The compound premodifier as a typologically incompatible syntactic pattern

The use of premodifying adjectives instead of verbose post-modifying noun complements is a popular technique of compression, as shown by the *electric* example. The use of compound premodifiers in English terms is generally a stylistic choice, but it is not readily transferrable to typologically distinct languages, such as Polish.

---

[2] For English it has been argued that the non-head of a compound does not require a syntactic category, but in inflectional languages such as Polish, even base forms of same-stem words representing different word classes are different from each other. In this example, *włącz* and *wyłącz* are evidently imperative forms in the 2nd person singular.

The English compound premodifier (such as *logic-defying* in *logic-defying theories*) is a compressed form of the adjectival/participial phrase complement of nouns ([*theories*] *defying logic*), which in turn is a compressed version of the relative clause postmodifier ([*theories*] *that defy logic*). Note that there is no compression of meaning, since even if the corresponding post-modifying adjectival complement includes a prepositional phrase (*specific to mice* ⇒ *mouse-specific*), the missing preposition is readily retrieved by the reader during text comprehension since deletion of the preposition has a systematic nature (i.e. it applies to all constructions of this type).[3] The compound pre-modifier is quite frequently used to create terms in the same way as *cigarette smoking* is more academic than *smoking cigarettes*.

Compare *sulphate-reducing bacteria*, the Polish equivalent of which is our first example in this section, and *bacteria reducing sulphates*. The latter phrase can be interpreted as a descriptive one, perhaps naming a property of several groups of bacteria, while the premodified version is a term. In Polish, the word order is freer and more sequences of three words are felicitous (*bakterie redukujące siarczany*, *redukujące siarczany bakterie*). As stated before, post-modification of a head noun makes a phrase term-like. However, participial modifiers in LGP are usually also placed to the right of nouns and so the phrase in question is still perceived as a non-restrictive descriptive phrase. The Polish language lacks a good equivalent of the definite article in the generic meaning it has as an element of terms. In English, it is the use of a definite article together with the particular word order that accounts for the term-like appearance of phrases with compound premodifiers, while *bacteria reducing sulphates* will be understood as a descriptive phrase. In Polish, the term is rendered as *bakterie redukujące siarczany*, but it is normally preceded by *tzw.* ('so-called'), indicating that the phrase is not term-like in Polish.[4] Another rendition is the abbreviation *SRB*.

---

[3] Cases where the head adjective or noun governs different prepositions are rare, and many compound premodifiers are derived from phrases that do not include prepositions, e.g. *coffee-grinding machine*. The singular vs. plural uncertainty is also resolved: the nouns are usually plural because scientific statements apply to groups (mice) rather than individuals (a mouse) and so the reading is 'all individuals of a given type of objects'.

[4] Pearson (1998) listed the phrase *so-called* as a signal that could be used to identify terms in texts written for the general audience or for students, but she did not detect the same pattern of use in texts for other specialists (the *Nature* corpus) (Pearson 1998:127, 131).

The second example is the compound adjective *press-fit*, which describes a type of hip joint implant. It was used in a Polish article in (7).

(7) stosowanie ciasno dopasowanego przeszczepu tzw. *press-fit* ('the use of a tightly fitted implant, so-called press-fit').

The difficulty lies in translating the sense of 'press-fit', i.e. fitted by pressing. The phrase 'tightly-fitted' in the sentence fragment refers to the same activity, but sounds like a descriptive phrase (note the pre-modifier position in Polish) describing a potentially gradable trait as if an implant could be fitted with more or less slack. The use of this phrase as a component of the Polish equivalent of the term *press-fit implant* would amount to a semantic extension, or rather narrowing, of the LGP phrase *tightly fitted*, so that it would specifically refer to the process of fitting this kind of implant. In English, the terminological character of this three-word whole is signalled by structural means, i.e. the compound pre-modifier.

Interestingly, the term *press-fit* was not coined for medical purposes. It has been taken over from the language of technology, where its Polish equivalent, as given in a dictionary, is *pasowanie wtłaczane* (lit. 'fitting$_N$ pressed', i.e. pressed fitting). The author of the sentence quoted above might not have known that an equivalent existed, but let us also note that, if it was decided to translate *press-fit,* it would not be possible to turn the participle *wtłaczane* into an adverb so that it could modify the participial equivalent of *fit*.

The two examples show that the rendition in Polish of compound pre-modifiers as components of English terms causes difficulties similar to those encountered in the case of metaphorical terms: their word-for-word equivalents are marked as unnatural or the terms are rendered as abbreviations or loanwords.

7 Non-analytical terms: culturally-determined preference levels?

While languages for specific purposes have been defined as language varieties that are learned together with their concept systems (Cabré 1999: 65) rather than acquired in early childhood, they can still be claimed to have their 'native speakers', in the sense that field experts, who are their primary users, store the special knowledge of their fields in their minds (Grucza 2008: 137). With this paper, I have tried to account for an unwillingness on the part of Polish medical doctors and medical scientists, who, in accordance with the above statement, are the most competent individuals to use medical terminology, to adopt word-for-word translations of certain types of English medical terms. The adoption of LGP words as metaphorical terms by English-language LSP users and the avoidance of this naming technique in terminology by Polish authors alludes to the existence of a stylistic rift between an 'Anglo-Saxon' and a 'Teutonic' style with regard to LSP texts (see e.g. Duszak 1994). The presence of English borrowings in Polish medical texts should not be ascribed entirely to the dominance of English as a lingua franca in science. Many borrowings represent structures that are difficult to reproduce syntactically in Polish and calqued metaphorical terms are usually accompanied by signals of their alien nature (the phrase *so-called* or quotation marks) or the original terms in brackets. Abbreviations also tend to be used instead of full terms that are difficult to render in Polish. According to this conceptualisation, the borrowing of medical terms is a sign of the inability to render certain types of compression or typologically dissimilar patterns of term formation and an unwillingness towards accepting terms derived in a way that is incompatible with terminological traditions in Poland. Overall, the phenomena in question paint a picture of typological and culture-related differences between national terminologies and possibly shed new light on the borrowing of English terms into other languages.

References

Amchikunga.com (no date), 'Tibetan Medicine', http://www.amchikunga.com/Services.html (viewed 12 June 2014).

Cabré, Maria Teresa (1999), *Terminology: theory, methods, and applications,* Amsterdam: John Benjamins Publishing.

Duszak, Anna (1994), 'Styl teutoński, czyli o tworzeniu barier komunikacyjnych' [The Teutonic style or the creation of barriers to communication], in Gajda, Stanisław & Nocoń, Jolanta (eds.), *Kształcenie porozumiewania się: materiały konferencji naukowej, Opole 26-28.09.1994,* Opole: Uniwersytet Opolski, 257-264.

EJO = Polański, Kazimierz (ed.) (1999), *Encyklopedia językoznawstwa ogólnego* [Encyclopaedia of general linguistics], Wrocław: Ossolineum.

Felber, Helmut & Budin, Gerhard (1989), *Terminologie in Theorie und Praxis* [Terminology in theory and practice], Tübingen: Gunter Narr Verlag.

genenames.org (no date), 'Symbol Report: CXCL8', http://www.genenames.org/cgi-bin/gene_symbol_report?hgnc_id=6025 (viewed 15 June 2014).

Gilreath, Charles T. (1995), 'Resolving Term Disputes with Weighted Onometrics', in Wright, Sue Ellen & Strehlow, Allan (eds.), *Standardizing and Harmonizing Terminology: Theory and Practice, ASTM STP 1223*, Philadelphia: American Society for Testing and Materials, 25-52.

Górnicz, Mariusz (1997), 'Sposoby i granice kompresji terminów (na podstawie terminologii medycznej – nazwy nowotworów)' [Methods of and limits to term compression (based on medical terminology – names of neoplasms)], *Poradnik Językowy* 2/541:25-32.

Grucza, Sambor (2008), *Lingwistyka języków specjalistycznych* [Linguistics of languages for specific purposes], Warszawa: Euro-Edukacja.

Guillén Galve, Ignacio (1998), 'The textual interplay of grammatical metaphor on the nominalizations occurring in written medical English', *Journal of Pragmatics* 30: 363-385.

ten Hacken, Pius (2008), 'Prototypes and Discreteness in Terminology', in Bernal, Elisenda & DeCesaris, Janet (eds.), *Proceedings of the XIII EURALEX International Congress*, Barcelona: Documenta Universitaria, 979-987.

Halliday, Michael A.K. (1994), *An introduction to Functional Grammar. Second Edition*, London: Arnold.

Ickovich, Victor A. (1972), 'Новые тенденции в образовании аббревиатур (О путях включения аббревиатур в систему языка)' [New tendencies in abbreviation formation (On the ways of incorporating abbreviations in the language system)], in Danilenko, Valeriya Petrovna (ed.), *Терминология и норма* [Terminology and norm], Moskwa: Nauka, 88-101.

ISO (2009), *ISO-704 2009 Terminology work - Principles and methods*, Geneva: ISO, http://www.iso.org/iso/catalogue_detail.htm?csnumber=38109

Jadacka, Hanna (1999), 'Zapożyczenia' [Borrowings], in Markowski, Andrzej (ed.), *Nowy słownik poprawnej polszczyzny* [New dictionary of Polish usage], Warszawa: Wydawnictwo Naukowe PWN, pp. 1773-1775.

LDOCE (2003), *Longman Dictionary of Contemporary English*, Summers, Donna (ed.), Harlow: Pearson Education.

Leitchik, Vladimir M. (1981), 'Оптимальная длина и оптимальная структура термина' [Optimal length and optimal structure of term], *ВОПРОСЫ ЯЗЫКОЗНАНИЯ* 2: 63-72.

Madycki, Grzegorz; Staszkiewicz, Walerian; Wycech, Agnieszka & Kuryłowicz, Michał (2004), 'Kinking tętnicy szyjnej wewnętrznej – ocena występowania, wskazania do zabiegu operacyjnego oraz ocena odległych wyników leczenia na podstawie wyników badań ultrasonograficznych' [Internal carotid artery kinking — actual incidence, indications for surgical treatment and long-term results based on ultrasound evaluation], *Chirurgia Polska* 6/4: 185-193.

Musiołek-Choiński, Karin (1986), *Polskie nazwy chorób. Studium z terminologii medycznej* [Polish names of diseases. A study in medical terminology], Wrocław: Wydawnictwo Uniwersytetu Wrocławskiego.

Pearson, Jennifer (1998), *Terms in Context*, Amsterdam: John Benjamins Publishing Company.

Sager, Juan C. (1990), *A practical course in terminology processing*, Amsterdam: John Benjamins Publishing Company.

STP (2005), *Języki specjalistyczne. Słownik terminologii przedmiotowej* [Languages for specific purposes. A dictionary of domain terminology], Lukszyn, Jerzy (ed.), Warszawa: KJS.

CHAPTER EIGHT

COMPOUNDING PROPERTIES AND TRANSLATION METHODS OF TERMS IN THE DOMAIN OF INFECTIOUS DISEASES

SZYMON MACHOWSKI

The research presented in this chapter belongs to medico-linguistics, a discipline located between medical sciences and linguistics. It is a modest contribution to a theory of word comparison in lingua medica (cf. Roberts (1953), Burnum (1997), Bettin and Gadebusch Bondio (2007) and Brooks (2008)). In particular, it will be devoted to the comparison of terms in the domain of infectious diseases in English and in Polish with respect to four onomasiological and four formational dimensions (parameters). The article consists of 6 sections. In section 1, the selection of English medical terms which appear as compound words is presented. They are analysed in section 2 and in section 3 the correlations between these compounds in terms of their onomasiological and formal properties are examined. After the methodology of analysis of the Polish translations of these terms has been presented in section 4, section 5 proceeds to the methods of translating English compounds into Polish. The latter analysis focuses at first on the dominating tendencies in compounding and next the minor tendencies are also given. In the final section 6, the results achieved have been briefly reviewed while focusing on similarities and differences prevailing in compounding being treated.

1 Sources and selection criteria of the English-language medical terms

Before the intended analysis proper, let me propose for consideration several general issues with the aim of justifying the necessity of the enquiry into the field under investigation here.

The analysed medical terms belong to the medicoprofessiolect. These terms as well as the other medicolingual terms deserve an in-depth linguistic analysis which can facilitate medicolingual communication within the medical community. This newly coined notion meets the following definition of a language community:

> A language community is a communicative community, which makes use of a uniform means of communication, that is, a common language. Hence, each language community is a communicative community but not conversely. The latter is a basis for the former. The language community can be viewed as a product of and a kind of superstructure imposed upon the corresponding communicative community. [Zabrocki (1963) as cited by Bańczerowski (2001: 37)]

The medical community can be conceived of as comprised of medical staff and medical patients irrespective of the appurtenance to their national or ethnic communities. The existence of such a community is in accordance with Zabrocki's (1963: 20) concept of overlapping social and occupational communities. As implied by his approach to the theory of communicative communities, both patients and hospital staff members simultaneously belong to various sociolinguistic groups, e.g. a physician can also be a grown-up offspring or a parent in their own family and as a consequence, they naturally use everyday expressions of their native language outside their jobs. Nevertheless, communication problems arise when patients contact health care system professionals, as indicated in reference books by such as Asher (1994: 1055-1057) and Crystal (2013: 402).

The need for an inquiry into medical communication was clearly recognized by Crystal (2013: 402) who wrote that "the field of medicine, more than any other, forces a confrontation between scientific and everyday language". One of the most common approaches to communication between medical professionals and patients, who are unfamiliar with medical jargon, is to make doctors ask their patients questions confined to the state of their body organs (Health 1979 as cited by Crystal 2013: 402). In the past, "patient-doctor language" (Asher 1994: 2433) was analysed from the pragmalinguistic point of view in terms of conversation analysis, language as a sequence of speech acts and language as a conversational cooperation (Asher 1994: 1055-1057). Asher also points out that the focus in the early 1990s was generally put on "Western medicine, particularly on American, British and German health systems" (Asher 1994: 1057). By contrast, this study also regards a few linguistic aspects of contemporary Polish medical discourse. The rapid increase in the knowledge about the underlying medical reality is also reflected in the terminology concerning diseases and technical equipment (Kloch 2013b: 51). Thus, contemporary medical staff, and physicians in particular, are made to develop another system of educating prospective physicians. The first signs of such a change have been reported in the United States, where medical students are to be taught to gain access to the specialist information they need (Kloch 2013a: 49).

Another reason for investigating the linguistic properties of the whole range of terminology related to infectious diseases in particular is an ongoing technological progress in producing vaccines which has recently resulted in having the citizens of the United Kingdom and the United States prevented from many common infectious diseases (see WHO 2012a). In turn, previously widespread infectious diseases in Poland, e.g. diphtheria, tetanus, whooping cough, mumps and German measles have now been prevented, especially among children and teenagers, thanks to the annually updated vaccination program (Mrukowicz, 2013). However, it seems to be significant to refer to some quite recent historical information on diagnosing and treating infectious diseases in Poland in order to present the current Polish medical vocabulary stock in a transparent way. A great amount of medical information closely related to the topic of this study might be found in several articles in English authored by Polish medical and laboratory staff (e.g. Służewski et al. 1999, Kowala-Piaskowska et al. 2004) which were accepted for presentation or publication in Western countries. Aside from their language, their issuing date also plays a crucial role because they were written before Poland's access to the European Union in 2004. Regarding linguistic aspects of the development of medical research on treating infectious diseases in Poland before 2004, it should be emphasized that the papers were very often written in English, which supports the statement that:

> English is now widely employed as a medium of instruction in medical schools in countries where it is a second or a foreign language. It is the main medium for medical textbooks, journals, and abstracting indexes, and is by far the most used language in international medical meetings [Asher (1994: 2432)] after Maher (1986).

Interestingly, Asher (1994: 2432) also mentions that "noun compounding is a common feature of medical terminology in some languages", which was also an incentive to linguistically explore medical terms within this research.

Contrary to most English-speaking countries and Poland, respiratory, blood and sexually transmitted infections are still very widespread in

Africa which is related to the poor economic condition of African countries (see WHO 2012b). The infections are frequently caused by numerous mutations of pathogens (see WHO 2012c). Therefore, my research is confined to the current lexis used by physicians in English-speaking countries and in Poland. Particular attention will be paid to current lexical methods used to give names to recently reported contagious pathogens and new medications in highly developed English native speaking and poor African countries. Noticeably, a large number of the new English-language lexical terms meet the definition of Bauer's (2000:695) English compound words. Interestingly, a number of them can be translated into the words or expressions representing a wide range of Polish grammatical structures other than Polish compound words, e.g. simple words and biconstituent or complex syntagms. Such observation has led to formulating the following principal research aims:

- to investigate the relationships between the English medical terms with respect to their onomasiological properties
- to analyse the grammatical structure of Polish equivalents of English medical terms.

The English-language lexical material is restricted to 140 medical terms as excerpted from the latest medical data provided by the World Health Organization and the issues of the *Journal of Infectious Diseases* from 2010 to 2013. As regards their linguistic properties, they have been approved if they meet the definition of an English compound word that is understood as "a lexical unit made up of two or more elements, each of which can function as a lexeme independent of the other(s) in other contexts" (Bauer 2000: 695).

2 Linguistic analysis of the English-language medical terms

The linguistic analysis of specialist compound words can be conducted along two dimensions, the onomasiological dimension and the formal dimension of word formation. With respect to the former, the four types in (1) can be distinguished.

(1) a. names of new forms of infectious microorganisms, e.g. *Ebola virus*, *A/H1N1 virus*

b. names of diseases, e.g. *Hydatid disease*, *Swine influenza A1H1*, *Herpes simples infection*, *Epstein-Barr-virus infection*, *HPV infection*
c. names of procedures of clinical diagnostics, e.g. *biotyping*, *biomonitoring*, *immunofluoresence*, *tissue culture*
d. names of newly elaborated pharmacological treatments, e.g. *lopinavir, telaprevir, ceftaroline, fidaxomicin, telavancin*

Proceeding to the latter dimension, the analysis of the compound words is based on their formational structure, in particular, the degree of their morphological connection (Bańczerowski 2008: 253) which to my mind finds reflection in their orthographic shape. The four categories listed in (2) can also be distinguished.

(2) a. open compounds with separately written components
b. hyphenated compounds whose components are linked by a hyphen
c. solid compounds are orthographically continuous without any hyphen or intermediate space
d. neoclassical compounds

In the medical vocabulary investigated, English open compounds (or appositional syntagms) can be exemplified by *complement fixation, Norwalk agent*, *tissue culture*, hyphenated compounds by *RT-PCR*, solid compound words by *histoplasma*, *smallpox*, *cowpox*, *chickenpox* and neoclassical compounds (2d) (cf. ten Hacken 1994, 2012), e.g. *immunosuppression*, *immunoblotting* and *immonofluorescence.*

The categories (2a-c) are mentioned by Lieber & Štekauer (2009: 7), although they do not consider the contrast between them crucial.[1] For (2a), we also find the term *appositional structure* (e.g. Sadler & Nordlinger, 2006), which suggests an analysis in which they are not treated as compounds. For (2d), Scalise & Bisetto (2009: 47) suggest that they are a subtype of subordinate compounds. Ten Hacken & Petropoulou (2002: 170) propose that they involve neoclassical formatives which are "available for the formation of new lexemes but they are not lexemes themselves, which implies that they are bound morphemes".

[1] There are also numerous cases in which the same compound may be written as an open or a solid compound. Thus, the COCA corpus (http://corpus.byu.edu/coca/) gives 120 occurrences of *chickenpox* and 237 of *chicken pox*.

3 Correlation between the onomasiological and formal properties of compounds

As already mentioned above, each compound word from the subset of the English medical professiolect treated here might be characterized by associating one of the biparametric types to this compound. These types are created by combining the values of the onomasiological and formal parameters listed in (1) and (2). Each such type will consist of the set of the theoretical sum of the corresponding two categories specified by these two dimensions (parameters).

As a result, the 140 medical terms in my sample are classified into the 16 biparametric types. These types have been associated with the corresponding symbols, e.g. indicating 1a2a – open compounds designating names of new forms of infectious micro organisms, 1b2a indicating open compounds designating names of diseases, etc. Table 8-1 gives examples for some of these types.

	2a	*2b*	*2c*	*2d*
1a	Ebola virus	-	-	flaviovirus
1b	Hookworm infection	Q-fever	chickenpox	campylobacteriosis
1c	PCR method	-	-	chromatography
1d	-	-	-	antiretrovirals

Table 8-1: Examples of selected classes

It is shown in Table 8-1 that the medical compounds from the 140-word sample fall into nine types out of the 16 theoretically possible types. This does not mean that the seven remaining ones do not exist, but they are not represented in the investigated sample. Therefore, the 16 potential types are not exhausted in the sense that in the sample no representatives were found for seven types.

It seems worth considering a method to create new compound words by means of blending (contamination). This operation has been investigated by Algeo (1977), Cannon (1986, 2000) and Hamans (2010, 2014). Hamans (2010, 2014) dealt with this operation in the domain of simple words. This operation as a function associates a word being a product of the blending with a pair of words from which it is obtained, e.g. (*motor*, *hotel*): *motel* (Hamans 2010: 463), (*Cambridge*, *Oxford*): *Oxbridge* (Hamans 2010: 456). We can extend this method of formation by contamination to compound words. That is to say that from a pair of words a new compound can be gained. Some examples appear in (3)

(3) a. (retroplasma, mycovirus): retrovirus
b. (mycovirus, cytoplasma): mycoplasma

The compound *retrovirus* has been borrowed from English into Polish. We could even speak of borrowing the operation of contamination and consequently a kind of English-Polish interlingual analogy commends itself which can be exemplified as follows: (*retroplasma*, *mycovirus*): *retrovirus* = (*retroplazma*, *mykowirus*): *retrowirus*. Obviously, this kind of analogy may operate intralingually too. However, it should be observed that, thus far, this method of compounding by contamination has been applied to a minor extent. Nevertheless, it can be viewed as a potential for prospective enriching of the set of compound words.

Unfortunately, the morphological structure of such compounds as *boceprevir*, *lopinavir*, *ritonavir* or *telaprevir* is not transparent and it requires further investigation. The examples of the above contaminated compounds all belong to the domain of neoclassical compounds. I am convinced that the domain of neoclassical compounds may turn out to be a rich reservoir for contaminated compounds in the future. This might be explained by the fact that neoclassical constituents (e.g. *allo-*, *morpho-*, *webo-*, cf. ten Hacken 2012: 84) are prone to be easily incorporated to the word formation structures of medical terminology and "can … appear in first or in second position" (ten Hacken 2012: 81). In addition, the analysis of the names of currently prescribed antibiotics has shown that neoclassical constituents may be active components of at least one productive blending operation. Therefore, the process of neoclassical word formation can possibly go together with blending by direct analogy to blending among simple words (as defined by Hamans, 2010: 457).

4 Methodology of analysing the Polish translation equivalents

Although the contrast between the open vs. solid structure and hyphenated spelling of compound words is generally rejected in English linguistics as a basis for recognizing compound words (e.g. Lieber & Stekauer 2009: 7), it is used in language books for hospital staff (e.g. Allum 2012). As opposed to these orthographic contrasts, neoclassical compounding is not only an English-language phenomenon (ten Hacken 2012: 78), but it "occurs in many European languages" (Panocová 2012: 31). Therefore, the incorporation of neoclassical constituents can be also assumed to be a productive word formation operation in Polish to coin specialist terms. This consideration was partly reflected in the analysis of the susceptibility of Polish and English medical compound words to blending. The most significant obstacle that hampers the comparative study seems to be found in mutually unsuitable English and Slavic grammatical approaches. This serious linguistic problem was mentioned for instance by Kavka (2014) and by ten Hacken (2013: 98), who refers to Dressler (2006: 24), as a difficulty in formulating a universal definition of compound words.

In this research, the aim is to develop a set of common methodological devices to investigate both Polish and English complex morphological structures in the medical professiolects. Hence, the above presented English categories have been tentatively applied to Polish vocabulary. The only exception has been made to open compounds which do not exist in Polish (e.g. Handke 1976: 10-12). It is implied by an obligatorily continuous linear compound structure in Polish (e.g. Handke 1976: 12). As a consequence, English open compounds have no direct Polish counterparts. Additionally, Polish compounds as translation equivalents will be analysed in terms of their morphological cohesion grade: high (HIGH) or low (LOW). It is absolutely necessary to emphasize that the general concept of morphological cohesion for contrastive purposes is opposed to Handke's (1976) and Bzdęga's (1985) contributions to the theory of compound cohesion in Polish and German (Bzdęga 1985), which are in turn based on the semantic equivalence between the compound constituents and the words in the corresponding syntagms. The alternative definition of compound cohesion seems to be sufficiently motivated by a strong need to find parallel representations of each cohesion type among both Polish and English medical terms. On the contrary, the traditional definition of a compound word in Polish linguistics, e.g. Urbańczyk and Kucała (1999: 452), Handke (1976: 10-12), is generally compatible with the ones adopted in German linguistics, by e.g. Eichinger (2000: 115) and Ortner (1984: 11, 14-16).

In this Polish and English contrastive study, the term "high morphological cohesion" is a property of the relation between the constituents of a compound which has a different meaning than the corresponding syntagm, e.g. *hookworm – worm of hooks*. On the other hand, "low morphological cohesion" is defined as a property of the relation between the constituents of a compound which has a very similar meaning to the corresponding syntagm, e.g. *ELISA method – method of ELISA*. It seems to be very remarkable that all the neoclassical (as defined by ten Hacken (1994, 2012) and Panocová (2012)) and non-neoclassical solid compound words from the analysed medical vocabulary have a high morphological cohesion grade of their constituents. The first group includes e.g. *toksokaroza* ('toxocarosis') *toksoplazmoza* ('toxoplasmosis') and the latter one *tęgoryjec* ('hookworm infection'), respectively. In *tęgoryjec* we have *tęgi* ('hard') and *ryj* ('snout') with the suffix *-ec* which creates a synthetic compound designating both the animal ('hookworm') and the infection. This concept of morphological cohesion grade seems to be related to the compound types defined by Matthews (2007). A considerable group of English non-neoclassical compound words of high morphological cohesion grade, e.g. *smallpox*, *cowpox*, *monkeypox,* seemingly correspond to root compounds described as compounds "formed without an affix, hence especially, in English, one which does not parallel a verbal construction" (Matthews 2007: 350). On the other hand, the vast majority of the analysed compounds, including all neoclassical ones and selected non-neoclassical solid ones, e.g. *tęgoryjec* ('hookworm'), tend to reflect the structure of synthetic compounds defined as compound words "derived with an affix; especially in English, one which parallels a verbal construction" (Matthews 2007: 398).

As mentioned in the introduction, English multi-word compounds are frequently translated into Polish syntagms (cf. Szymanek 2009: 466). In the set of examples considered here, all of the Polish syntagms have a determinative structure, which means they have determinators and determinata (cf. Bańczerowski et al. 1982: 244-257).

In order to approximate the structure of medical terms appearing in the form of syntagms, we can avail ourselves of the following syntagmatic types:

- rectional syntagms (Bańczerowski 1988: 1159-1182) or case government (Bańczerowski et al. 1982: 244-257) (C)
- agreement syntagms (Bańczerowski 1997a: 53-69) (A)
- multideterminational chains defined as "set of lexes which can be determinatively ordered in a sequence" (Bańczerowski 1980:90) (polyconstituent syntagms, PCS).

Syntagms can be exemplified by *choroba grypopodobna* ('parainfluenza'), *dur rzekomy* ('paratyphoid fever'), rectional syntagms by *metoda immunoblot* ('immunoblotting'), *borelioza z Lyme* (lit. 'disease of Lyme'), multideterminational syntagms by *zakażenie wirusem HIV* (lit. 'infection by HIV virus'), *wirusowe zapalenie wątroby typu A* (lit. 'virus inflammation of the liver type A') and *wirusowe zapalenie wątroby typu B* (lit. 'virus inflammation of the liver type B').

The Polish translation equivalents have been excerpted from Polish articles on bacteriology and virology from issues of *Nowiny Lekarskie* ('Journal of Medical Science'), *Przegląd Epidemiologiczny* ('Epidemiological Review') and *Medycyna Praktyczna – Szczepienia* ('Practical Medicine – Vaccines') from 2010 to 2013. Importantly, the focus is exclusively put on the English compounds which have Polish counterparts in the medical press. This method is illustrated in Table 8-2.

compound word being a medical term	***biparametric type***	***Polish equivalent***	***typology of the Polish equivalent***
Kawasaki disease	1b2a	choroba Kawasaki	C
chickenpox	1b2c	ospa wietrzna	A
campylobacteriosis	1b2d	kampylobakterioza	2d (HIGH)
PCR method	1c2a	metoda PCR	C
Rotarix vaccine	1c2a	szczepionka Rotarix	C
ELIZA method	1c2c	metoda ELIZA	C
antiretrovirals	1d2d	przeciwretrowirusowy	2d (HIGH)
telaprevir	1d2d	telaprewir	2d (HIGH)

Table 8-2: Examples of English compounds and their correspondences with their Polish equivalent types

The above table presents the method of correlating biparametric English compound types with their Polish equivalents of various grammatical structure. As exemplified in the second column, the biparametric English compound types are formed by correlating the onomasiological and word formation properties of the analysed compound words. In turn, the Polish translation equivalents (column 4) are described by the symbols which stand for their respective grammatical types: compound types (2d) or syntagms (A, C, PCS). This aims at giving an insight into the type of correlation in question.

5 Methods of translating English compounds into Polish

Another key goal is to suggest and discuss ways of translating English compound words into Polish. Since the methods are restricted to the vocabulary of infectious diseases and their treatment, they are presented as major (dominating in other words) or minor translation tendencies in terms of their (moderately) high or low frequency. This classification is based on the above linguistic terminology. Additionally, each tendency is illustrated in a series of tables.

5.1 Three dominating tendencies

Once all the English-Polish translation pairs were analysed, it was possible to identify the most numerous group, which covers 93% of translations among the medical vocabulary investigated. This group illustrates the translation methods which also seem to be generally most representative and highly productive in the English-Polish translation of compound medical terms. The first of these tendencies is closely related to the analogical word formation structure of mutual neoclassical translation equivalents and to the inclusion of onomasiological constituents (or words) to the structure of English and Polish compound words (see Table 8-3).

compound word being a medical term	*bipara-metric type*	*Polish equivalent*	*typology of the Polish equivalent*
cytomegalovirus	1a2d	cytomegalovirus	2d (HIGH)
histoplasmosis	1a2d	histoplazmoza	2d (HIGH)
mononucleosis	1b2d	mononukleoza	2d (HIGH)
mycobacteriosis	1b2d	mykobakterioza	2d (HIGH)
toxocariasis	1b2d	toksokaroza	2d (HIGH)
autolysin	1c2d	autolisina	2d (HIGH)
biomonitoring	1c2d	biomonitorowanie	2d (HIGH)
chemotherapy	1c2d	chemioterapia	2d (HIGH)
chromatograhy	1c2d	chromatografia	2d (HIGH)
electrophoresis	1c2d	elektroforeza	2d (HIGH)
immunofluorescence	1c2d	immunofluorescencja	2d (HIGH)
spectography	1c2d	spektografia	2d (HIGH)
ultrasonography	1c2d	ultrasonografia	2d (HIGH)
antiretroviral	1d2d	przeciwretrowirusowy	2d (HIGH)
boceprevir	1d2d	boceprevir	2d (HIGH)
ceftaroline	1d2d	ceftarolina	2d (HIGH)
simeprevir	1d2d	simeprevir	2d (HIGH)
telaprevir	1d2d	telaprewir	2d (HIGH)
telavancin	1d2d	telawancyna	2d (HIGH)

Table 8-3: Examples where an English neoclassical compound is translated into a Polish neoclassical compound

Based on the examples given in Table 8-3, the analysed English and Polish neoclassical compound words explicitly show structural and semantic similarities and their constituents correspond with each other in terms of their meaning and their position in the linear structure of compounds. Moreover, it is impossible to associate them with any equivalent syntagm which they might possibly come from according to Bzdęga's (1985) concept. The Polish and English neoclassical terms might be almost literally translated in both ways. Because of their solid structure, native speakers probably feel the higher degree of what Bańczerowski (2008: 253) calls *morphological connection* than in hyphenated compounds. As noted about the semantic properties of the entire set of neoclassical compound words investigated in English and in Polish, the initial constituents determine the final ones, e.g. in *ultrasonography ultra-* determines *-sonography* or in *toxocariasis toxo-* determine *-cariasis*. A different group of cases is represented in Table 8-4.

compound word being a medical term	***bipara-metric type***	***Polish equivalent***	***typology of the Polish equivalent***
Lyme disease (Lyme borreliosis)	1a2a	borelioza z Lyme	C
Herpes simplex infections	1a2a	zakażenie wirusami z rodziny Herpesviridae	PCS
paratyphoid fever	1b2a	dur brzuszny	A
tapeworm infection	1b2a	tasiemczyca tkankowa	A
Lassa disease	1b2a	choroba Lassa	C
foodborne botulism	1b2a	zatrucie jadem kiełbasianym	PCS
CNS imaging	1c2a	badanie obrazowe	A
FluBlok vaccine	1c2a	szczepionka FluBlok	C
Norwalk agent	1c2a	czynnik Norwalk	C
PCR method	1c2a	metoda PCR	C
Rotarix vaccine	1c2a	szczepionka Rotarix	C
tissue culture	1c2a	hodowla tkanek	C
Tzanka test	1c2a	test Tzanka	C
complement fixation	1c2a	odczyn wiązania dopełniacza	PCS

Table 8-4: Examples where an English open compound designating an illness, a clinical procedure or a pathogen into a Polish biconstituent syntagm (A, C) or a determination chain (PCS).

The analysis of the group of English compounds in Table 8-4 should be divided into two subgroups which could be called an operation of syntagmatization. The first subgroup consists of very few open compounds (or appositional syntagms) such as *complement fixation* or *foodborne botulism* that can be translated into Polish expressions that have the structure of syntagms. Another subgroup exemplifies a rather numerous set of English open compounds (or appositional syntagms) that are regularly translated into Polish expressions that have the structure of agreement or rectional syntagms. In many cases the order of the constituents in the English compounds is reversed in the word order of the corresponding Polish syntagms, e.g. *Norwalk agent – czynnik Norwalk, Lyme borreliosis – borelioza z Lyme, PCR method – metoda PCR, Rotarix vaccine – szczepionka Rotarix.* This statement might be particularly true for the English and Polish constructions that have a constituent designating a proper name which is either a brand name of any chemical substance, e.g. *FluBlok PCR*, *Rotarix* or an inventor's or producer's own name, e.g. *Tzanka* or a place name, e.g. *Lyme*, *Lassa*. Nevertheless, the determinative structure of the English open compounds (or appositional syntagms) is analogous in the Polish translations. The third tendency is illustrated in Table 8-5.

compound word being a medical term	*biparametric types*	*Polish equivalent*	*typology of the Polish equivalents*
chickenpox	1b2c	ospa wietrzna	A
cosackievirus	1a2c	wirus Cosackie	C
mumpsvirus	1a2c	wirus świnki	C

Table 8-5: Examples where an English solid compound is translated into a Polish biconstituent syntagm

As shown in Table 8-5, English solid (non-neoclassical) compound words tend to be translated into Polish biconstituent expressions that have the structure of agreement or rection syntagms. Only one explicit regularity might be observed. If an English solid compound includes a constituent that designates a proper name, e.g. *Cosackie*, it is regularly translated into a Polish expression that has the structure of a bicomponential rectional syntagm. The order of words in the syntagm is reversed to the order of their corresponding constituents in English. As regards the comparison between the two tendencies in Table 8-4 and 8-5, a significant difference might be found in the structure of the English compound words translated into Polish syntagms only. These compound words can be either of open (see Table 8-4) or solid non-neoclassical structure (see Table 8-5). In turn, agreement and rection types of syntagms may be distinguished.

To summarize the presentation of the dominating tendencies, it seems inevitable that all English and Polish neoclassical compounds represent the same morphological scheme. In compound words in both languages neoclassical constituents (as defined by e.g. ten Hacken (2012)) are bound morphemes according to the definition by Elson and Pickett (1968: 6). In turn, English open biconstituent compounds or two-word appositional syntagms are likely to have a Polish equivalent which is an agreement or rection syntagm. The compound constituents tend to convey the same meaning as their Polish counterpart words in the syntagms. This statement is generally true for the biconstituent ones. As for open compound words (or alternatively complex appositional syntagms) with three or more constituents, they are generally translated into Polish as expressions representing complex syntagms. Thirdly, English solid compounds predominantly correspond with Polish biconstituent agreement or rection syntagms. Similarly to the open ones, the vast majority of the words of their Polish translation equivalents tend to convey the same meaning as their corresponding compound constituents in English. Another curiosity of the Polish and English non-neoclassical solid compound words is the possibility to classify them as non-lexicalized compounds (or alternatively *Zusammenrückungen*) (Bussmann 2008:766) because they have "flexion markers" (Bussmann 2008:766) in their inner structure, e.g. *mumpsvirus*.

5.2 Three minor tendencies

In direct reference to the dominating tendencies, the minor translation tendencies cover 7% of all the translation pairs. They were grouped and presented in order to present the grammatical phomenana which are rarely made of the Polish-English translation of medical compounds. The translation tendencies are also related to the very low frequency of onomasiological and grammatical structures in the investigated vocabulary. For these tendencies, the tables give all the examples in the corpus. A first group is presented in Table 8-6.

compound word being a medical term	***biparametric types***	***Polish equivalent***	***typology of the Polish equivalents***
cowpox	1b2c	krowianka	SIMPLEX
tuberculosis	1b2c	gruźlica	SIMPLEX

Table 8-6: Examples where an English solid compound is translated into a Polish simple word

Table 8-6 represents a very limited number of English solid compound words that are translated into Polish simplex words. An important property of this type of English compounds is their morphological connection (in Bańczerowski's terms). As mentioned above, the meaning of these compounds has been relexicalized in comparison to the corresponding paraphrase, e.g. *cowpox – pox of cows*. A second minor group is represented in Table 8-7.

compound word being a medical term	*biparametric types*	*Polish equivalent*	*typology of the Polish equivalents*
Borrelia infection	1b2a	borelioza	SIMPLEX
Denge fever	1b2a	denga	SIMPLEX
Hydatid disease	1b2a	bąblowiec	SIMPLEX
scarlet fever	1b2a	ornitoza	SIMPLEX
Yersinia infection	1b2a	jersinioza	SIMPLEX

Table 8-7: Examples where an English open compound is translated into a Polish simple word

The most striking feature of this minor translation tendency seems to be the predominant role of the initial constituents of the English open compounds (or appositional syntagms) in the English-Polish translation process in the sense that the form of the Polish equivalents that have the structure of simple words is directly semantically related to just the initial constituents in their English counterparts. This tendency is particularly easily observable if an English constituent has onomasiological properties, i.e. conveys the meaning of an internationally recognized sickness, e.g. *Borrelia*, *Denge* and *Yersinia*. Finally, there is one example of a further translation strategy, given in Table 8-8.

compound word being a medical term	*biparametric types*	*Polish equivalent*	*typology of the Polish equivalents*
Q-fever	1b2b	gorączka Q	C

Table 8-8: Example where an English hyphenated compound is translated into a Polish syntagm

Table 8-8 illustrates an English compound word representing an extremely limited class of hyphenated medical compounds represented by only one compound in the corpus investigated. They have an onomasiological constituent and are likely to be translated into Polish biconstituent expressions that have the structure of rection syntagms.

On the basis of these examples, some minor generalizations can be formulated. Firstly, Polish simplex morphological constructions tend to be quite frequent translation equivalents of several rarely occurring and usually highly cohesive English solid and open compound words. What is more, the small number of hyphenated tokens in the vocabulary investigated might be implied by the rare use of hyphens in American English (cf. Peters 2004, Allum 2012). This variety of English was the language of the main excerption sources used in the research, such as the *Journal of Infectious Diseases*.

6 Concluding remarks

To conclude, the analysis of medical vocabulary in the domain of infectious diseases shows that English solid compounds tend to be neoclassical. The possibility to form compounds by means of contamination (blending) has not been fully implemented thus far. Moreover, a number of English neoclassical compounds can be almost literally translated into Polish using highly cohesive compounds, which is in accordance with their high productivity in creating new words in European languages (e.g. ten Hacken 2012, Panocová 2012). In this case, both current English and Polish neoclassical compound words have parallel structures. In the corpus of English medical vocabulary I investigated, there are quite a numerous amount of representatives of solid or open compounds that mostly designate the various diseases. They are very often translated into Polish expressions which belong to syntagms, e.g. (agreement) syntagms or rection syntagms (case government).

References

Algeo, John (1977), 'Blends, a Structural and Systemic View', *American Speech* 52 1/2: 47-64.

Allum, Virginia (2012), 'English for Medical Purposes: Health Care Assistants', Raleigh, NC: Lulu.

Asher, R.E. (ed.) (1994), *The Encyclopedia of Language and Linguistics*, Amsterdam: Elsevier.

Bańczerowski, Jerzy (1980), *Systems of Semantic and Syntax*, Warszawa: Państwowe Wydawnictwo Naukowe.

—. (1988), 'A contribution to the theory of concord', in Basaj, Mieczysław & Borek, Henryk (eds.), *Wokół języka. Rozprawy i studia poświęcone pamięci Profesora Mieczysława Szymczaka*, Wrocław: Wydawnictwo Polskiej Akademii Nauk, 53-69.

—. (1997), 'A theory of rection', in Hickey, Raymond & Puppel, Stanisław (eds.), *Language History and Language Modelling: a Festschrift for Jacek Fisiak on His 60th Birthday*, Vol. 2, Berlin: Mouton de Gruyter, 1158-1182.

—. (2001), 'The linguistic legacy of Ludwik Zabrocki', in Puppel, Stanisław (ed.), *The Ludwik Zabrocki Memorial Lecture. Suprema lex: cognoscere, legere, disputare, docere*, Poznań: Adam Mickiewicz University Press, 9-51.

—. (2008), 'Wyraz w ujęciu morfologiczno-typologicznym' [A morphologico-typological approach to words] in Bednarczuk, Leszek; Smoczyński, Wojciech & Wojtyła-Świerzowska Maria (eds.), *Językoznawstwo historyczne i typologiczne. W 100-lecie urodzin Profesora Tadeusza Milewskiego*, Kraków: Polska Akademia Umiejętności, 233-259.

Bańczerowski, Jerzy; Pogonowski, Jerzy & Zgółka, Tadeusz (1982), *Wstęp do językoznawstwa* [Introduction to linguistics], Poznań: Adam Mickiewicz University Press.

Bauer, Laurie (2000), 'Compounding', in Haspelmath, Martin; König, Ekkehard; Oesterreicher, Wulf & Raible, Wolfgang (eds.), *Language Universals and Language Typology*, Berlin: Walter de Gruyter, 695-707.

Brooks, Stewart M (2008), *Lingua Medica: Everyone's Guide To Understanding Medical Terminology*, Beaverton: Ringgold Inc.

Burnum, John F. (1997), 'Lingua medica. A physician's Hamlet', *Annals of internal medicine* 126 (5): 412-414.

Bussmann, Hadmoud (2008), *Lexikon der Sprachwissenschaft* [Lexicon of Linguistics], Stuttgart: Kröner.

Bzdęga, Andrzej (1985), 'Zusammenbildungen in der deutschen und polnischen Gegenwartssprache', *Glottodidactica* 17: 31-39.

Cannon, Garland (1986), 'Blends in English word formation', *Linguistics* 24:725-753.

Cannon, Garland (2000), 'Blending', in Booij, Geert E.; Lehmann, Christian; Mugdan, Joachim & Skopeteas, Stavros (eds.), *Morphologie: Ein Internationales Handbuch Zur Flexion und Wortbildung,* Berlin: Walter de Gruyter, 952-956.

Crystal, David (2013), *The Cambridge Encyclopedia of Language. Third edition*, Cambridge: Cambridge University Press.

Dressler, Wolfgang. U. (2006), 'Compound Types', in Libben, Gary & Jarema, Gonia (eds.), *The Representation and Processing of Compound Words*, Oxford: Oxford University Press, 23-44.

Eichinger, Ludwig (2000), *Deutsche Wortbildung. Eine Einführung*, Tübingen: Günter Narr Verlag.

Elson, Benjamin. F. & Pickett, Velma B. (1968), *Beginning Morphology and Syntax*, Dallas: SIL International.

Gadebusch Bondio, Mariacarla & Bettin, Hartmut (2007), *Lingua Medica: Lehrbuch zur medizinischen und zahnmedizinischen Terminologie*, Berlin: Logos Verlag.

ten Hacken, Pius (1994), *Defining Morphology: A Principled Approach to Determining the Boundaries of Compounding, Derivation and Inflection*, Hildesheim: Olms.

—. (2012), 'Neoclassical Word Formation in English and the Organization of the Lexicon', in Gavriilidou, Zoe; Efthymiou, Angeliki; Thomadaki, Evangelia; Kambakis-Vougiouklis, Penelope (eds.), *Selected Papers of the 10th International Conference of Greek Linguistics*, Komotini: Democritus University of Thrace, 78-88.

—. (2013), 'Compounds in English, in French, in Polish, and in General', *SKASE Journal of Theoretical Linguistics* 10: 97-113.

ten Hacken, Pius & Petropoulou, Evanthia (2002), 'Neo-classical word formation in WM electronic dictionaries', in Braasch, Anna & Povlsen, Claus (eds.), *Proceedings of the Tenth EURALEX International Congress* EURALEX 2002, Copenhagen, 169-174.

Hamans, Camiel (2010), 'The productivity of blending: Linguistic or cognitive? Or how to deal with administrativia and ostalgia', in Stanulewicz, Danuta; Wolański, Taduesz Z. & Redzimska, Joanna (eds.), *Lingua Terra Cognita II. A Festschrift for Professor Roman Kalisz*, Gdańsk: Wydawnictwo Uniwersytetu Gdańskiego, 467-490.

—. (2014), 'What makes a blend – a Reading Report and Some Observations', in Kleparski, Grzegorz; Konieczna, Ewa; Kopecka, Beata (eds.), *Linguistics and Methodology. The Subcarpathian Studies in English language, Language and Culture*, Rzeszów: Wydawnictwo Uniwersytetu Rzeszowskiego, 240-256.

Handke, Kwiryna (1976), *Budowa morfologiczna i funkcje compositów polskich (z uwzględnieniem innych języków zachodniosłowańskich)* [The Morphological construction and function of Polish compound words (with regard to other West Slavic languages)], Warsaw: Zakład Narodowy im. Ossolińskich.

Heath, Shirley Brice (1979), 'The context of professional languages: an historical overview', in Alatis, James, E. (ed.), *Language in Public Life*, Washington, D.C.: Georgetown University Press, 102-118.

Kavka, Stanislav (2014). 'Can we arrive at an agreement on the compound status?', paper presented at the 12th Conference of the European Society for the Study of English, Košice, 29 August - 2 September 2014.

Kloch, Agnieszka (2013a), 'We should teach medical students to ask questions and seek answers', *AKADEMIA. The magazine of the Polish Academy of Sciences* 4 (40):49.

—. (2013b), 'Working together to revitalize the physician-scientist workforce of tomorrow', *AKADEMIA. The magazine of the Polish Academy of Sciences* 4 (40):50-51.

Kowala-Piaskowska, Arleta; Mozer-Lisewska, Iwona; Figlerowicz, Magdalena; Machowska, Ludomiła & Służewski, Wojciech (2004), 'Interleukin 6 and 12, Alanine Aminotransferase Activity, and HCV Viral Load in Children with Chronic Hepatitis C Treated with Interferon and Ribavirin', *Inflammation* 28(6):319-325.

Lieber, Rochelle & Štekauer, Pavol (2009), 'Introduction: Status and definition of compounding', in Lieber, Rochelle & Štekauer, Pavol (eds.), *The Oxford Handbook of Compounding*, Oxford: Oxford University Press, 3-18.

Maher, John C. (1986), 'The role of English as an international language of medicine', *Applied Linguistics* 7: 41-52.

Matthews, Peter H. (2007), *The Concise Oxford Dictionary of Linguistics*, 2nd Edition, Oxford: Oxford University Press.

Mrukowicz, Jacek (2013), 'Program szczepień ochronnych w Polsce na 2013 rok – co nowego?' [The program of preventive vaccination in Poland in 2013 – what is new?], http://www.mp.pl/pediatria/artykuly-wytyczne/wytyczne/show.html?id=79269 (viewed 29 Nov. 2014).

Ortner, Hanspeter & Ortner, Lorelies (1984), *Zur Theorie und Praxis der Kompositaforschung*, Tübingen: Gunter Narr Verlag Tübingen.

Panocová, Renáta (2012), 'Morphological properties of neoclassical formations in English', *Bulletin of the Transilvania University of Brasov. Philology and Cultural Studies* 5 (54) 2: 31-36.

Peters, Pam (2004), *The Cambridge Guide to English Usage,* Cambridge: Cambridge University Press.

Roberts, Ffrangcon (1953), 'Lingua medica. A study in medical semantics'. *British Medical Journal* 1: 1444-1447.

Sadler, Louisa & Nordlinger, Rachel (2006), 'Apposition as coordination. Evidence from Australian languages', in Butt, Miriam & King, Tracy Holloway (eds.), *Proceedings of the LFG06 Conference*, Stanford: CSLI Publications, 437-454.

Scalise, Sergio & Bisetto Antonietta (2009), 'The classification of compounds', in Lieber, Rochelle & Štekauer, Pavol (eds.), *The Oxford Handbook Of Compounding*, Oxford: Oxford University Press, 34-53.

Służewski, Wojciech; Figlerowicz, Magdalena & Machowska, Ludomiła (1999), 'Influence of endo- and exogenous interferon-α on the course and treatment of chronic hepatitis B in children', paper presented at the conference Immunology and Liver. Basel, 20-21 October.

Szymanek, Bogdan (2009), 'IE Slavonic: Polish', in Lieber, Rochelle & Štekauer, Pavol (eds.), *The Oxford Handbook of Compounding*, Oxford: Oxford University Press, 34-53.

Urbańczyk, Stanisław & Kucała, Marian (eds.), (1999), *Encyklopedia języka polskiego* [Encyclopedia of the Polish Language], Wrocław: Zakład Narodowy im. Ossolińskich.

Zabrocki, Ludwik (1963), *Wspólnoty komunikatywne w genezie i rozwoju języka niemieckiego 1. Prehistoria języka niemieckiego* [Communicative communities in the genesis and development of the German language, Vol. 1, Prehistory of the German language], Wrocław: Zakład Narodowy Ossolińskich.

Appendix: Sources of Corpus Data

Journal of Infectious Diseases, 201 (1-12), 202 (1 -12), 203 (1-12), 204 (1-12), 205 (1-12), 206 (1-12), 207 (1-12), 208 (1-12). Arlington: Infectious Diseases Society of America.

Journal of Medical Science (previously *Nowiny Lekarskie*) (2010-2013), 79 (1-6), 80 (1-6), 81 (1-6), 82 (1-6), Poznań: Poznań University of Medical Sciences. http://www.nowinylekarskie.ump.edu.pl/ (viewed 29 Nov. 2014).

Medycyna Praktyczna – Szczepienia [Practical Medicine – Vaccines] (2010-2013), http://www.mp.pl/szczepienia/ (viewed 2. Nov. 2014).

Przegląd Epidemiologiczny [Epidemiological Review] (2010-2013), 64 (1-4), 65 (1-4), 66 (1-4), 67 (1-4).
http://www.pzh.gov.pl/przeglad_epimed/ (viewed 29.Nov.2014).

WHO (2012a), 'World Health Organization Global Advisory Committee on Vaccine Safety, report of meeting held 5 to 6 December 2012', http://www.who.int/vaccine_safety/committee/reports/Dec_2012/en/ (viewed 11 Nov. 2014).

WHO (2012b), 'World Health Organization Global Report for Research on Infectious Diseases of Poverty 2012', http://whqlibdoc.who.int/publications/2012/9789241564489_eng.pdf?ua=1 (viewed 4 Nov. 2014).

WHO (2012c), 'World Health Organization Influenza virus activity in the world 14 September 2012', http://www.who.int/influenza/gisrs_laboratory/updates/summaryreport_20120914/en/ (viewed 4 Nov. 2014).

LIST OF CONTRIBUTORS

Rachel Bryan, Swansea University

María Fernández Parra, Swansea University

Mariusz Górnicz, University of Warsaw

Pius ten Hacken, Leopold-Franzens-Universität Innsbruck

Pilar León-Araúz, University of Granada

Szymon Machowski, Adam Mickiewicz University, Poznań

Renáta Panocová, Pavol Jozef Šafárik University in Košice

Nina Patton, Swansea University

Sevda Pekcoşkun, Kırklareli University

Rocío Pérez Tattam, Swansea University

AUTHOR INDEX

Subject Index